# THE
# BEAUTIFUL GAME
### AND THE
# UGLY TRUTH

# THE
# BEAUTIFUL GAME
## AND THE
# UGLY TRUTH

### Football's Tragic Link with Dementia
#### Foreword by Chris Sutton

K I E R A N   G I L L

First published by Pitch Publishing, 2022

Pitch Publishing
9 Donnington Park,
85 Birdham Road,
Chichester,
West Sussex,
PO20 7AJ
www.pitchpublishing.co.uk
info@pitchpublishing.co.uk

A CIP catalogue record is available for this book
from the British Library.

ISBN 978 1 80150 118 7

Typesetting and origination by Pitch Publishing
Printed and bound in India by Replika Press Pvt. Ltd.

# Contents

# Acknowledgements

THANK YOU Jemma. In my two years of writing this book, we bought our first home, acquired our first dog (Arya the cockapoo), got engaged and entered our 30s, all amid a pandemic. I couldn't have wished for a better partner throughout this entire process.

Thank you to my mam, Audrey, my dad, John, my sister, Alison, my brother-in-law, Joe, and my nana, Joan, for allowing me to mention my grandad, Robert, who we lost to dementia in 2017.

Thank you to the Cameron-Barr-Henderson clan, Martin, Julie, Joss, Daisy, Liam, Belle and Indie.

Thank you to Jane Camillin and Pitch Publishing for your faith and patience.

Thank you to Marc Padgett and the *Daily Mail* for permitting me to work on this project.

Thank you to the campaigners, including Chris Sutton, Dawn Astle, John Stiles, Dr Judith Gates, Penny Watson and Katherine Snedaker, and the researchers, Professor Willie Stewart, Dr Ann McKee and Chris Nowinski, and my colleagues, such as Mike Keegan, Sam Peters, Jeremy Wilson and Andy Bull, for your work in this field which proved invaluable.

Finally, with each copy sold I will make a donation to a dementia charity, so thank you for reading.

# Foreword by Chris Sutton

*Premier League winner and son of Mike, former professional footballer who died with dementia*

CHANCES ARE you know – or knew – someone with dementia and have had the displeasure of seeing what this disease can do to a human being. It isn't merely little lapses in memory. Like that time you lost your car keys, or misplaced your mobile phone, or drew a blank when trying to think of the name of that friend you've known for donkey's. We can laugh at those mishaps, those 'oh, what are you like' moments. Then it escalates. Then it's not so harmless. Then you comprehend what a cruel master it can be. There is no cure for dementia; once it's got its claws into you, it never lets go. It's a daily deterioration, stripping you of your memories, your dignity, the lot.

Dementia stole my dad, Mike, from me. He was a proud man. Strong, funny, sharp. Then after a decade-long decline, he succumbed, on his own and in a care home we weren't allowed to visit due to Covid-19 restrictions. We hoped he could spend his final days at his home in Horsford, Norwich, where he had lived with my mum, Josephine, since 1974. Unfortunately that wasn't allowed. He was so fragile that he needed 24-hour specialist care. By the time the full-time whistle was blown, at the age of 76 and on 26 December 2020, my dad was a shell of the man he once was. Unable to walk, his last six months were spent horizontal, lying in bed. He was medicated to the teeth, in an adult nappy and so confused. He couldn't converse when we visited – when lockdown let us, that is – and it was a bleak existence by the end. It was no way to go. Nobody's dad, mum, grandmother, grandpa, brother or sister deserves to die in such an undignified way.

My dad was a former professional footballer. What's that got to do with dementia, you ask? Well, everything. He headed ball after ball and I believe that is ultimately what killed him. He died with dementia – specifically something called Chronic Traumatic Encephalopathy, which you may recognise better as CTE. I remember my dad telling me how, at Norwich City, he and his team-mates would head medicine balls in training – the idea being that it would strengthen their neck muscles. Imagine! What madness. Research by Professor Willie Stewart at Glasgow University has now proven that ex-players are at a greater risk of dying with neurodegenerative disease than the man in the street. As a former footballer myself – and someone who headed tens of thousands of balls over the course of my career – that's scary.

I miss my dad. I don't have closure. What I do have is a nagging feeling in the pit of my stomach – one which tells me that football, the game he loved and I love, killed him and is still killing others today. That's what's so sad in all of this. It's still happening and it'll continue to happen until football's authorities do something about it. Personally, I'd like to see protocols introduced to protect current and future generations, such as compulsory heading restrictions in training, and temporary concussion substitutions in games. I don't see the harm in either of those, but still we wait for the game to get off its backside. There's been a great deal of denial, not unlike the tobacco industry's refusal to recognise that smoking cigarettes causes cancer, and that's alarming. Like I told the MPs when I was invited to give evidence on the sorry situation in football, there is blood on the hands of those who have done and continue to do nothing.

I know the author of this book well. I know Kieran has witnessed dementia in all its despair within his own family and I know, like me, he's passionate about this problem. I have the utmost respect for him for writing this book. It was needed to expose football's arrogance and its dismal attitude towards brain damage. Had I known about all this when I was a professional player, I would have done things differently. I wouldn't have headed 100 balls a week in training. Not a chance. I can't take that back now. It's too late for me, and it's too late for my dad. But it's not too late for football to make changes that could, literally, save lives. Enough is enough.

# Introduction

# 'A Football Disease'

*Jimmy Robson, Robert Rowland and millions of
others playing a game of cognitive Russian roulette*

'THE BALL would disappear up in the sky and when it
came down, I'd head it. There's more than me that's got this
problem, you know?' Those were the words of Jimmy Robson
in a chat kindly arranged by his daughter, Dany, towards
the end of 2020. Jimmy had become the seventh member of
Burnley's 1959/60 First Division title-winning side to develop
dementia. The other six had died but he was here, alive if not
still kicking, sitting in his favourite armchair, a Costa coffee
warming his hands. Dany had warned I might not get much
out of Jimmy. His memory fails him most days. You could try
asking about 16 December 1961 – how he married Beryl on
the morning at St Stephen's Church then faced Arsenal in the
afternoon at Turf Moor, supporters showering him in confetti
as he walked out of the tunnel. But it's unlikely he'd recall it
with any real clarity.

Sometimes the lapses in memory make you cry. Other times
laugh. When Nobby Stiles was announced as the latest footballer
to die with dementia, Dany asked her father what he thought of
it all. 'It makes me very sad because I might end up getting it,
too,' he replied, unaware he'd been under its spell for the last five
years. Today is a good day, though. Today the fog has cleared.

Today Jimmy can tell me what it was like to be a footballer and a very good one at that.

Mention of old team-mates' names sets Jimmy on a trip down memory lane and for a moment, this 81-year-old's human limitations seemingly melt away. He talks about Burnley being a solid footballing side. About Jimmy McIlroy being their best player. About scoring for fun alongside strike partner Ray Pointer. 'Oh we were good,' he says, wearing a cheeky smile. It's a disease-defying moment and one Dany puts down to a trip to Turf Moor, the home of his beloved Burnley, on the eve of our conversation. 'There was a big picture of the title-winning team in the *Burnley Express* newspaper,' she explains. 'Dad was asking us, "Am I on that?" There was no recognition there. But when we took him to Turf Moor and showed him a picture of the team, he could name all of them. Being there brought it all back for him.' Jimmy is not only aware of his own diagnosis on the day we speak. He is lucid enough to recognise the regrettable presence of dementia in the professional game. 'It is a football disease,' he says, simply but significantly. As the last survivor of the Burnley seven, he'd attended enough funerals of former team-mates to know.

Jimmy moved into the Wordsworth House Residential and Dementia Care Home in Hapton eight months after our conversation, a deterioration taking him to a point of no return. The Robson family had previously received some financial support from the players' union but, bizarrely, that stopped the moment Jimmy moved into his new £3,600-a-month home. The game looked the other way. The Robsons were on their own and it was on the wintry morning of 14 December 2021 that Jimmy passed away, aged 82. At 1.50pm on 29 December he was driven past Turf Moor one last time while on his way to St Stephen's. Here in body but not in mind for the final chapter of his life, Jimmy's was a tale familiar to many families, my own included.

Robert Rowland worked on the coal face at Horden Colliery in County Durham. He started there at the age of 14 but he was good at football; so good that First Division Burnley invited him for a trial at 16 after a scout spotted him during a Saturday kick-about. Robert never got to take up that invitation because his mum, Elizabeth, said he had to remain home and be an 'earner' for the family. Doing as he was told, he stayed in Horden and spent his days on his hands and knees, in dirt and dust, crawling in tunnels 1,200ft underneath the North Sea.

It was a dangerous job. The occasional injury inflicted by a falling rock kept Robert from the football field, with one such cave-in leaving him requiring surgery on his left ankle. But the field was where he spent his spare time otherwise, with the other local lads, a ball and time to kill in between shifts down the shaft. He played daily and took the whacks all footballers do, from goalkeepers to goalscorers. You will not find a Wikipedia page for Robert, who lived then died with dementia on 20 February 2017. While I like the idea of him sharing a changing room with Jimmy at Burnley in an alternative universe, he never got paid to play football in reality. But it was through Robert that I first discovered what dementia can do to a person. He was my grandad – the man who seemed so indestructible in my youth and yet was destroyed by this insidious disease of the mind. As anyone familiar with dementia will know, it's a slow death, and a long goodbye.

I've known Jimmy Robson, a champion of the professional game who scored the 100th FA Cup final goal at Wembley Stadium in 1962. And I've loved Robert Rowland, an amateur who graced the local grass and treated Horden green as if it was his own Wembley. As Chris Sutton wrote in his foreword, chances are you've known someone with dementia, too. Perhaps a relative who never pulled on a pair of boots. Maybe someone who didn't head a ball in his or her life. It can invade men and women in any walk of life, though its presence among former footballers is clear. It's come for enough to suggest players are playing cognitive Russian roulette.

Some we've lost. Others we're still losing. From Jeff Astle to Alan Jarvis, Joe Mercer to Ernie Moss, Mike Sutton to Nobby Stiles, Dave Watson to Jimmy Hill, Denis Law to Wim Jansen, Joe Kinnear to Sue Lopez, Gordon McQueen to Rod Taylor. Six players from Aston Villa's 1957 FA Cup-winning side are said to have succumbed to such problems, along with four from Tottenham Hotspur's Double-winning team of 1961 and seven from Manchester United's 1968 European Cup-winning squad. The deterioration of England's World Cup winners of 1966 is evidence that dementia doesn't discriminate. It doesn't give a damn about your name or your achievements, whether you're Jack Charlton or Sir Bobby Charlton, Bertie Auld or Hilderaldo Bellini, Bob Paisley or Danny Blanchflower, Ferenc Puskás or Gerd Müller.

Throughout this book, I will refer to former footballers by their first names. They aren't just players; surnames on the back of shirts. They're human beings, and it's important to remember that when considering the consequences which can come with playing the world's most popular sport.

What follows is largely a story of failure. It's the Football Association, Premier League, Professional Footballers' Association and world governing body FIFA knowing about a potential problem for decades. It's 'Mr Blackburn Rovers' Tony Parkes relying on fan-led crowdfunding to cover £4,000-a-month home care costs – another man neglected by the multi-billion-pound industry he served so well. It's the dismissive attitude towards Chronic Traumatic Encephalopathy, the degenerative brain disease found in those with a history of repetitive head trauma, footballers included. It's the controversy surrounding the concussion protocols and those who set them. It's the perpetual insistence that 'more research' is required – the game's little escape clause. It's the inaccuracies about why footballers of today need not worry about forgetting their own names in the future because, apparently, this is a problem of the past. It isn't. This is the beautiful game and its ugly truth. This is football and its tragic link with dementia.

# 1

# A History of 'Punch-Drunk' Players

*Football's custodians cannot say they weren't
warned amid a century of cautionary tales*

ON 4 August 1939, the former captain of Manchester United, Charlie Roberts, was sitting in a private room at Manchester Royal Infirmary. With him was a reporter from the *Daily Mirror*. 'They have found a growth at the back of my skull which has developed as a result of heading heavy balls so often over 20 years ago and are going to extract it,' said the 56-year-old retired centre-half. 'I have been almost like the living dead for the last two years, especially after my active life.' Charlie's chronic dizziness and headaches had alarmed specialists who said he needed surgery. 'When I was told I was to have an operation I refused point blank,' continued Charlie. 'But when I thought it over I decided that anything was better than going on as I have for the last two years.'

Three days after speaking to the *Mirror*, Charlie was dead. Those paying a penny for a copy of the next day's newspaper would read the ex-England international's parting words, spoken prior to him entering surgery. 'A month in here and a few weeks' holiday, then I will be able to go and see United play again.' He lived for football, then he died for it, his doctors said.

Cases could be made for Roy Keane, Bryan Robson and a few others as the club's greatest captain. Hardly anyone can say they surpassed the achievements of Charlie, however. He is right up there in the pantheon of United greats, a leader of leaders and man with morals. Signed from Grimsby Town for £600 in 1904, he captained United to their maiden First Division titles in 1908 and 1911 and FA Cup glory in 1909. Yet away from the crunching tackles, terrific clearances and exhilarating evenings at Bank Street and then Old Trafford – that stadium switch coming midway through Charlie's time at the club – he was an equally powerful force off the pitch.

With United colleague Billy Meredith, he co-founded the players' union, known today as the Professional Footballers' Association. It followed a footballing tragedy when their team-mate Tommy Blackstock died during a reserve game against St Helens Recreation in the Manchester suburb of Clayton on 8 April 1907. Reports say the 25-year-old from Kirkcaldy headed the ball close to the halfway line, collapsed and never got back up. A sturdy Scottish defender whose desire to deny opposition strikers was so strong, it was written he would 'go at a stone wall if the stone wall seemed likely to score a goal'. Yet as touching as these tributes were to Tommy, hailing his fearlessness and dedication, the Blackstock family received nothing in compensation. That appalled Charlie and so he sprang into action, almost as quickly as he would to clear a cross.

At the Imperial Hotel in Manchester on 2 December 1907, Charlie chaired the union's first meeting. He complained about footballers dying and families left destitute, about the Football Association and their cap on wages. Although it cost him his England career – no caps followed after picking this fight with the FA – Charlie won in the end. Today's PFA exists, in no small part, thanks to this pioneer. The union celebrate that fact, too. In 2015 they spent £30,000 at auction to secure the shirt he wore in United's 1909 FA Cup Final win. That's £30,000 more than was spent on investigating football's link to dementia that same year, and the year after, and the year after that. Research, which would finally provide answers, started in 2018 with the PFA funding it to the tune of £125,000. Good news, at last, though the game's custodians have long been accused of looking the other way when the warnings were there in black and white and in front of them.

Headaches have been making headlines for more than a century. There were red flags before Charlie Roberts and the seven-and-a-half-hour operation on his brain and many more raised after. Surveying a century of clippings from newspapers and magazines, sifting through papers provided by researchers, speaking to historians who specialise in the subject of neurology – you soon realise football's dark relationship with brain damage wasn't exactly hidden.

In the *Lincolnshire Echo* on 16 September 1903, for example, was a report about Sam Nicholls, the former West Bromwich Albion centre-forward who was in a serious condition at Queen's Hospital, Birmingham. 'He is suffering from an affection of the brain and this is the persistency with which he used to head the ball. Doctors say that the practice is fraught with considerable danger,' the newspaper said. Also reporting on the health of Sam, who scored in the 1892 FA Cup Final, the *Barnsley Chronicle* wrote, 'This is one of the great drawbacks of the association game, the practice being unquestionably dangerous.' In the *Northern Daily Telegraph* on 14 April 1910 was a story about a 16-year-old called Walter Truelove who played a match on the Saturday, complained of a headache on the Sunday then passed away on the Monday. 'Continually heading the ball whilst playing football would cause the condition,' read the report, mentioning he died with acute meningitis. 'A fall on his head would also do so.' And then there's the article in the *Burnley Express* on 28 February 1931 about a 24-year-old called Horace Harrison who headed for goal, staggered to the sideline and then collapsed. He died, and a doctor told an inquest into his death that it is 'extremely dangerous to head a heavy wet ball' because it can have 'the effect of sandbagging'.

Just a few examples. It's easy to fall down a rabbit hole of research once you get going. Players have died on the pitch after freak accidents. John Thomson was the supremely talented 22-year-old Celtic goalkeeper kicked in the head by Rangers striker Sam English on 5 September 1931, dying later that same day. It occurred in front of 80,000 supporters at Ibrox and 40,000 crammed into the small Scottish town of Cardenden, Fife, for his funeral. His Celtic team-mates carried his coffin from his home on Balgreggie Road to Bowhill Cemetery. Hundreds climbed on to the roofs of houses for a better view, their caps removed from their heads and pressed against their chests as John passed by. Such fatal accidents aren't common in football, thankfully. Death by dementia is, however, and one headline of old is direct and to the point. 'Football's corridors awash with punch-drunk former players' it declares, with *The Guardian* likewise pondering 'punch-drunkenness' among footballers in a piece published on 28 November 1969.

The term 'punch-drunk' was coined in a paper published in the *Journal of the American Medical Association* in 1928 by an American pathologist called Dr Harrison Martland. It talked about prize fighters feeling the consequences of considerable head punishment and how boxers were also derided as 'cuckoo', 'goofy' and 'slap happy', among other crude terms. Champion boxer Del Fontaine – real name Raymond Henry Bousquet – was hanged on 29 October 1935, convicted of shooting and killing his 21-year-old girlfriend Hilda Meek in a jealous rage over a phone call about a late-night rendezvous with another man. Naturally the newspapers were all over this case, publishing the police statement taken at the scene of the crime in Kennington, south London. 'She has broken my heart and ruined my life,' the attending officers were apparently told. 'She had her fortune told by a gypsy some time ago, who said she would be murdered in three years. I said, "My God, never," and to think I should be the one to murder her.'

His defence was described as one of the most unusual ever heard in the Old Bailey as it was claimed the Canadian had a 'confused brain' and was 'so punch-drunk as a result of his fights that he could not have known the nature of his act'. He had fought north of 100 fights in his career and taken some batterings. His last bout in Newcastle did not even last a round. 'Bousquet was knocked down three times,' read one report. 'The third time the back of his head struck the floor violently.' Witnesses were called to explain their experience of his 'punch-drunkenness' in court. Boxing manager David Edgar described it as a 'vacant look, far-away thoughts, and general unbalance'. Welterweight world champion Ted 'Kid' Lewis said he had seen this affliction in plenty of his peers, adding the accused had endured 'more punishment' than anyone else he had ever seen.

Though alarm bells were ringing about how regularly this boxer's bell had been rung, the insanity defence didn't wash with the jury. They took only half an hour in their deliberations to find him guilty of murder and Del Fontaine was duly sentenced to death at Wandsworth Prison. A petition containing more than 20,000 signatures was presented to the Home Office three days before his hanging, but it was dismissed. There would be no reprieve; no saving this former fighter from the rope and scaffold. 'They have hanged an insane man,' said the anti-capital punishment activist Violet Van der Elst, leading a protest on the morning of his passing outside Wandsworth.

It was two years after the conclusion of the Del Fontaine case that the less derisive term 'dementia pugilistica' was introduced to replace 'punchy' and those other primitive expressions – some of which were made in reference to boxers in Martin Scorsese's

1980 film *Raging Bull*, starring Robert De Niro as the troubled Jake LaMotta. Today it's more commonly known as Chronic Traumatic Encephalopathy, or CTE. Currently it is a disease which can only be diagnosed after death, by dissecting the brain and analysing what lies beneath the surface. The symptoms in those suspected of living with the condition vary. It isn't simply forgetfulness. It's fits of rage. It's paranoia. It's depression and suicidal thoughts. It's piercing headaches and Parkinsonism. It's dementia, and it's been reported in footballers, boxers, American footballers, rugby players, even a 33-year-old circus clown who was repeatedly fired out of a cannon. Those who share a history of blows to the head, in other words, both concussive and subconcussive.

Some in the scientific community warn it is a condition still in its infancy, with lots to learn about who gets it, who doesn't and why. 'Contrary to common perception,' explained an editorial in *The Lancet* in 2019, 'the clinical syndrome of CTE has not yet been fully defined, its prevalence is unknown, and the neuropathological diagnostic criteria are no more than preliminary.' Others say there is more than enough evidence of its presence in contact sports.

Whether 'punch-drunk' or 'dementia pugilistica' or CTE, there is proof of this affliction causing concern over the last century. Not only among those who throw and take punches for a living but those who would put on a pair of boots and pull up their socks for our entertainment each Saturday. 'You don't have to go into the boxing ring and get one on the point for the K.O. to become punch-drunk,' readers of the *Gloucester Citizen* were told on 9 November 1944. 'You may quite as easily achieve this undesirable condition at football.'

In the season before the 1966 World Cup, supporters could pick up a copy of *Soccer Review*. Over the next decade this journal of the Football League would become a big hit. At its peak it's said to have enjoyed a circulation of 350,000 and early editions indicate this magazine was trying to highlight a growing issue in the game. One copy from November 1965 carries a 'GIVES EM HEADACHES' headline on its front cover. Former Leeds United footballer-turned-journalist Tom Holley is the author. 'As an old centre-half in league soccer,' he writes, 'I can simply report that I have suffered countless headaches from head work, let alone concussion. Most players have. And still do, but how many punch-drunk footballers have been reported?'

In October 1966, the same magazine, now renamed *Football League Review*, carries a column by Harry Brown with the headline 'DANGER IN HEADING THE BALL?' The write-up explains how boxing is not the only sport in which 'punch-drunks' can be found. 'Time and again after a game I suffer from headaches, obviously from all the heading I do,' says Derek Dougan, the Leicester City forward. 'I never had headaches before I started playing, and I've never really got rid of them,' adds Tom Holley. Apparently Tommy Lawton – described by his England colleague Sir Stanley Matthews as the 'greatest header of the ball I ever saw' – suffered from the same problem, while Everton goal machine Dixie Dean always carried aspirins with him. An unnamed club medical officer is unsure whether heading the ball is to blame but he does say, 'Continual jarring of the brain tissue could and does affect players sometimes.'

And there you have it. Another warning, scarcely two months after England's greatest achievement in football. Harry concludes his column by pondering why more isn't being done in light of these 'punch-drunks' in professional football. 'Couldn't club doctors get together and find out just what there is in it?' It is a column which would not look out of place in newspapers today, asking pertinent questions and wishing for answers. Harry doesn't mention dementia but it is clear he is making a connection between football and traumatic brain injury and calling for consideration. It is crying out for research, much like an article which appeared in the *Sunday Times* on 3 November 1974 under the headline 'Head Damage'. It was about a group of footballers whose deaths had been linked to the game. 'The figures represent an extreme minority of the millions who play football,' *Times* readers were told. 'But death from heading happens. Why? Medical research into heading is as thin as bone china.'

Perhaps the most extraordinary article I've encountered is from 1984 and entitled 'How Dangerous Is Heading?' It is remarkable because it is proof that world governing body FIFA have known about a potential problem for decades. We know this because the article was published in *FIFA Magazine*, their own publication. It raises the possibility of CTE. It insists the only immediate protection would be to decrease heading. It warns footballers are becoming concussed in training without realising it. It highlights players whose deaths were potentially provoked by football. It details a 1925 incident in which a 20-year-old developed a headache and dizziness during a game before losing consciousness and dying from 'subdural hematoma' – a bleed on the brain. 'The sports medicine community has not devoted enough attention to this important problem of possible brain damage,' concludes the article, authored by Vojin Smodlaka. 'When an athlete is knocked down and is unconscious for several seconds during a competition, in many cases he or she will be allowed to immediately continue the game – but if an athlete sustains a sprain or strain, he or she will stop. The sports community must take brain concussions more seriously.'

Chris Sutton started his professional career with Norwich City in 1991, seven years after this piece was published. 'It's astonishing,' he says. 'A major problem was flagged in their own magazine and yet what was done to protect players like me? I headed the ball day in, day out. We all did. And yet here, in black and white and in 1984, the dangers were being highlighted. It makes me wonder how many people from my generation will end up suffering, and how many of those were preventable, had action been taken. I've got a lump in my throat thinking about that.'

In response to the discovery of this article, the governing body defended their track record. 'FIFA takes its responsibility in relation to the topic of brain injuries very seriously as protecting the health of players is – and will remain – a top priority in developing the game,' said a spokesperson.

Nice words, but then this write-up was presented to FIFA's medical committee at a meeting in Zurich on 26 October 1984. Maybe they're dedicating more time to this problem today, now that it's been confirmed footballers carry a heightened risk of dementia compared to the general population. As the authorities in charge of the global game, though, it was the warning which appeared in their own publication in 1984 which players like Chris wishes FIFA had acted upon.

It was not only in newspapers and magazines that red flags were raised about the rising risk of brain damage. They also appeared in medical journals and the like, both home and abroad. In 1933, the *National Collegiate Athletic Association medical handbook for schools and colleges* warned that 'concussion of the brain' and 'fracture of the skull' are not only terms reserved for car accidents. They warrant special attention in sport, too. 'The seriousness of these injuries is often overlooked,' it warned, while insisting concussion should be defined as 'bruising of brain tissues' to underline its severity. This handbook was to be used by the doctors, coaches and trainers of athletic squads to provide the best care possible or, as the NCAA put it, prove 'helpful in the administration of their responsibility'. Decades later this document would crop up as American football was gripped by accusations that those in charge shirked this responsibility.

'There is definitely a condition described as "punch-drunk",' the handbook added.

In 1962, an article appeared in the German medical journal *Deutsche Medizinische Wochenschrift* with the title 'Über Verletzungen des Nervensystems beim Fußballspiel', translated as 'Injuries to the Nervous System when playing Soccer'. That study was highlighted at a 1968 conference in the United States with attendees hearing there was an 'increasing number of neurologic injuries from soccer due to propelling the ball with the head'. In 1972, an article appeared in the *British Medical Journal* called 'Footballer's Migraine', a term which players plagued by headaches would use among themselves in changing rooms. In 1980, another *BMJ* article called 'Serious Head Injury in Sport' was published, discussing cumulative damage in football and emphasising that it isn't only boxers who should be concerned about their careers.

In 1995, an article appeared in the *International Journal of Geriatric Psychiatry* called 'Are Professional Footballers at Risk of Developing Dementia?' It was prompted by the death of Tottenham Hotspur legend Danny Blanchflower at the age of 67. 'Preventative action could be taken by football's governing bodies to reduce the risk of brain damage as a result of head injury and subsequent development of dementia,' it summarised.

Norman Giller is the former Fleet Street sportswriter and author of more than 100 books. His 97th was *Danny Blanchflower: This WAS His Life*. For each copy sold, £5 went to the Tottenham Tribute Trust, the charity supporting former footballers in need, such as those struggling with the same condition which clouded Danny's mind. Norman recalls the time he went to interview the man who did the double with Tottenham in 1961, hoping for a nice, nostalgic, 30-year anniversary piece for the *Daily Express*. 'Danny and I had known each other well for years, but when I sat him down he did not know me from Adam, or Eve, for that matter,' he says. 'Worse still, he could not remember a thing about the First Division and FA Cup triumph or any of his team-mates. The most talkative and intelligent footballer I had ever known just looked at me blankly, his memory wiped clean. It was heartbreaking to see the game's great visionary with no knowledge of what he had achieved. Two years later he passed on at 67, unaware that he had been a football icon.'

This century of cautionary tales shows that dementia in football is by no means a new phenomenon, though it is now a much more recognised problem. It's in the mainstream. It crops up in conversation at the pub. It's circulated by campaigners on social media. It features on the back pages of newspapers who fight for justice. On 22 September 2013, led by Sam Peters, the *Mail on Sunday* launched a campaign after a series of high-profile concussion cases in rugby union. On 31 May 2016, led by Jeremy Wilson, the *Daily Telegraph* launched a campaign calling for sport to address its 'scandalous' neglect of research into dementia. On 17 November 2020, led by Mike Keegan, the *Daily Mail* launched its 'Enough is Enough' campaign, a powerful back page in black and white showing 28 former footballers diagnosed with dementia.

Clubs now treat this topic with the sensitivity it deserves. On 12 August 1995, at the annual meeting of the American Psychological Association in New York, attendees heard how a scientific survey had found footballers who frequently headed the ball scored significantly lower in IQ tests. The findings were widely reported and made their way to England. *The Times* contacted the authorities for comment, with the FA blaming it on 'years gone by, when the ball was made of leather, absorbed rain and became twice as heavy' in a statement. The newspaper also approached clubs. 'I don't think heading the ball has got anything to do with it,' quipped a spokesperson from an unnamed Premier League side. 'Footballers are stupid enough, anyway.'

Sometimes the families of former footballers can grow frustrated. Sometimes they feel the discussion can disappear and coverage wane. Then a familiar pattern will play out. A former player will have his condition made public and with that, dementia in football is a feature on the six o'clock news all over again. Denis Law, the former Manchester United man and only Scottish footballer to have won the Ballon d'Or, announced his diagnosis on 19 August 2021. Known previously as 'The King', 'The Lawman' and 'Denis the Menace' in his playing days, he became a broadcaster after hanging up his boots, renowned for his humour. That came across in his announcement. 'The time has come to tackle this head on, excuse the pun,' said the Scot too talented for only one nickname. Two days later, former Liverpool favourite Terry McDermott announced he had dementia, too. 'I'm not frightened of taking it on,' Terry said in his statement, 'and also, as we've seen, there are a lot of former players in a worse state than me.' Their reveals started up the conversation all over again – the one about how safe it is to play the world's most popular sport and what should be done. They were the latest warnings in a long history of them.

## 2

# 'Good Handwriting for a Doctor'

*The medical man who wanted to investigate in the*
*1990s but was patronised and ignored*

THE WARNING signs were there in black and white and for
sale on the shelves of newsagents. Reports there for reading.
Obituaries there for observation. Studies there for consideration.
The *Football League Review* column which highlighted the
potential consequences to playing the game coincided with a
notable First Division clash on the particular Saturday it was
published. Nottingham Forest triumphed 4-1 over title rivals
Manchester United that day, though that is no excuse for
ignoring the issue. Naturally then, there are sceptical sons and
dubious daughters and wives and widows of former footballers
diagnosed with dementia who are frustrated. They find it hard
to believe the folks in charge of English football were not aware
of the problems gripping their players, regardless of how busy
they were governing the game. Certainly it would be impossible
to plead ignorance to some warnings of old, such as those which
were sent directly to the Football Association, Premier League
and Professional Footballers' Association.

Dr John Rowlands was in contact with all three of those
organisations throughout the 1990s. He pleaded with them to
fund his research project. He told them he feared football had
a potentially deadly problem and that it needed investigating.

Now Dr Rowlands looks back in regret at how he was ignored. By them. By the clubs who didn't want to know. By the former players' associations who didn't want their members taking part in tests. In his possession is a treasure trove of evidence – three fat folders full of documents which, until now, were gathering dust in his garage. It's all there. The lousy letters from football's custodians. The decades-old handwritten notes. The newspaper cuttings as he tracked potential victims of playing the game, such as *The Journal* from 16 April 1998 in which north-east legend Bob Stokoe – the former Newcastle United centre-half and Sunderland manager – reveals how he suffers from a constant ringing in his ears. 'From the neck down I can't complain,' he says, 'but there is definitely something [that] happened to make my head bad and I think it was the headers.'

Dr Rowlands was first alerted to a potential problem through Norah Mercer. She was married to Joe, the Everton and Arsenal stalwart and legendary manager of Manchester City. Dr Rowlands was a family friend and GP in Liverpool. Norah had mentioned how many funerals she'd been attending of former footballers who lived then died with dementia. Too many to be a coincidence, she said. This was around 1980. Ten years later Norah would be attending her own husband's funeral. After a deterioration, Joe died on his 76th birthday on 9 August 1990. Some of football's most famous faces turned up at St Hildeburgh's Parish Church in Hoylake to pay tribute. 'Joe would have been pleased with the "gate" today,' joked Sir Tom Finney at the start of a stirring address. Another footballer dead after a dementia diagnosis, a headline in the *Daily Post* would later ponder the cause of Joe's demise, 'Did heading kill this man?' Dr Rowlands wanted to answer that question, or at least try. He was curious in a professional sense but also felt a personal responsibility. He had lost his friend and he wanted to help Norah.

With Dr Mark Doran, a consultant neurologist in Liverpool, a study was prepared which would 'determine the prevalence of dementia amongst professional footballers'. They posted this proposal to football's authorities and on the front cover was a quote from Brian Labone, the former Everton and England defender. 'We all know that we will die young or go mad,' it read. Dr Rowlands and Dr Doran planned to use the *Rothmans Football League Players Records – The Complete A–Z 1946–1981* to find the names of the 5,400 men, aged between 55 and 70, who had played football. They'd then contact each of these ex-players to conduct tests, known as 'The Telephone Interview for Cognitive Status'. The idea was this would enable them to detect how common dementia was in this group and compare it to the general public. They would also analyse the positions of the players to see how a goalkeeper, who hardly ever heads the ball, compares to a defender, who heads it aplenty. Initial estimations suggested the study would take one year to complete and cost a total of £73,000.

Dr Rowlands contacted the PFA and secured a meeting in Manchester with chief executive Gordon Taylor. The players' union promised to help but said he'd need to find funding to get his project off the ground. That is where he hit a series of brick walls, however, as his letters show.

There's one from the Medical Research Council in which he is told it is possible that professional footballers suffer from repetitive heading, rather like boxers from being punched. It's encouraging, until he's told it may be too difficult to conduct a study. Brick wall. There's another from the pharmaceutical company Pfizer in which Dr Rowlands is told if a link was made between footballers and Alzheimer's disease then this would have great implications on the game. However, with a promise that they will consider his proposal, he is then warned that funds are scarce. Months later they told him they could not support his study. Another brick wall.

Dr Rowlands wrote to the FA, and to the Premier League, and wasn't enthralled by either of their responses. He kept hold of those rejection letters. For legal reasons they cannot be reprinted in full in this book. However, we can discuss their condescending contents. The first letter is dated 15 July 1996 and from Graham Kelly, chief executive of the FA. Just two paragraphs long, it starts with a joke about how Dr Rowlands has got very good handwriting for a doctor and ends with a promise by Graham to consult the FA's medical department. Yet in another letter, dated 11 October 1996, it's clear no progress has been made. After being chased up by Dr Rowlands, Graham responds with a single paragraph, saying he'll ask the medical department again. You could file this under 'fobbed off'.

The Premier League weren't much more helpful. This ccompetition launched in 1992 would grow into a monster, feeding on the world's most talented footballers. Its pockets have always been deep, though all Dr Rowlands would get was the lint. He wrote to chief executive Rick Parry, who didn't bother replying himself. Instead the response came from Mike Foster, the Premier League's secretary, on 14 October 1996. Dr Rowlands is told there simply isn't the funds to back his project – but hey, here's an idea, why don't you ask the PFA?

Brick wall after brick wall. The idea was discussed at FA medical meetings but with no positive outcome for Dr Rowlands. He tried going to the clubs themselves and received a reply from one on 18 March 1996. The directors of this Premier League side had discussed it at their last board meeting but decided against helping, citing the enormous number of requests they receive for financial assistance. The chief executive of that club said he should try Gordon Taylor because he knew from a recent conversation with the PFA supremo that dementia in football was of concern to the players' union. Back to square one he went.

Dr Rowlands' local club, Liverpool, tried to help another way. They agreed to host a £45-a-head fundraising dinner at Anfield on 28 September 1996 with Jack Charlton – the former England footballer and Republic of Ireland manager who would later develop dementia – a guest speaker. It was in aid of the British Brain & Spine Foundation, who wanted to raise £250,000 to pay for research which could potentially protect future generations. They called their campaign 'NEURO 96', launching it in the same summer as that iconic tournament. Jimmy Hill, the distinguished broadcaster who was covering Euro '96 for the BBC and was later diagnosed with dementia himself, offered his support. 'Very positive,' reads one of Dr Rowlands' scribbled notes after a phone call with the punditry trailblazer who suggested they should try to organise a game with no heading.

Sadly the dinner at Anfield was cancelled, that trial match never arranged, and so they failed to secure the funding required. Football's reluctance to help its own frightened and frustrated Dr Rowlands, so he returned to the PFA. They had told him in their initial meeting that they would partially fund his project if he could find another backer. Now he wanted to know if they would be prepared to put their money on the table rather than wait for someone else to step in. The Premier League had said they provided the players' union with a 'substantial sum of money' each year for this sort of enterprise, after all, and it was now 1998. Years had passed since Dr Rowlands' first attempt at setting something up. At least if the PFA handed him their share of the funds then he could make a start. Maybe others would step in once he had started to produce results.

No such luck. He received a reply from Gordon Taylor on 27 April 1998. His letter began by mentioning the legal case in Scotland involving Billy McPhail and how it was adding to the conversation about dementia in football. Billy was the 70-year-old Glaswegian having his day in court. He was claiming that he deserved benefits, worth £70 a week, because heading the ball throughout his 17-year career had brought on his pre-senile dementia. He prided himself on his aerial ability. This was the centre-forward who scored a hat-trick of headers for Celtic in a 7-1 win over Rangers in the 1957 Scottish League Cup Final. Billy ultimately failed to convince the court that his job as a footballer was behind his suffering. In this letter, Gordon indicated he was watching the case with interest. He added that he was in contact with the FA's medical committee, who had agreed to place football's potential problem on their agenda.

A month later, Dr Rowlands was informed that a study taking in head injuries was now under way. It was an injury audit of the 1997/98 and 1998/99 seasons and being conducted in-house. This was arguably the biggest brick wall blocking Dr Rowlands' route to discovering the prevalence of dementia in football. He took it as a definitive sign that the FA did not want to use him to find out the truth and felt fobbed off. Distinctly little came of the study in terms of brain damage. It found there had been 6,030 injuries over the two seasons. The thigh accounted for 1,388 of those; the knee 1,014; the ankle 1,011. And so on. It broke down whether the injury was inflicted on the training ground or during a game. Whether it was while running, tackling, turning or stretching. Whether it was a muscular strain, fracture, tissue bruising or even a blister. It did not, however, tell us about neurodegenerative disease among former footballers. The word 'concussion' did not feature in the five-page report. Neither did 'dementia'. As good as it got was learning that 86 of the 6,030 injuries inflicted in this two-year period were to the head.

Dr Rowlands was out of ideas. Funding was never forthcoming for his own study and so nothing happened. 'I do regret that we didn't carry it through,' Dr Rowlands tells me. 'I do often wonder what might have happened, had we.' Taking part in a BBC Radio 5 Live special programme on dementia on 26 February 1998, former Liverpool defender and scout Geoff Twentyman discussed his diagnosis with him. 'I can still hear him,' says Dr Rowlands. 'He said, "I think it is the worst thing I have ever had in my life and I have had lots of complaints, but this Alzheimer's ..." and his voice gets slurred. I still think about that.' Several families who heard this programme wrote to the PFA to let them know of loved ones who were likewise living with the disease. Some of those letters were then forwarded on from the players' union to Dr Rowlands. He doesn't know why, 'On reflection, I am not sure what they thought I would, or could, do.' As the millennium approached, Dr Rowlands felt at a dead end. Every time he tried to make something happen, nothing did.

He was not the only one left with that deflated feeling. There were others who were likewise concerned and tried to alert the authorities. Dr Mike Sadler wrote to the PFA after noticing an alarming number of former footballers developing premature problems, including Bob Paisley. Some suspect this legend of Liverpool tried to compensate for his relatively small stature by playing through the pain, no matter how harsh a blow he suffered. Like on 30 October 1948, when he was apparently knocked unconscious in the first half against Newcastle United at St James' Park. 'During the interval the unusual method of walking him up and down outside the main grandstand was used in hope he would "come to",' revealed a report in the *Liverpool Evening Express*. He started the second half but didn't last. This was just one of many examples of machoism involving this great man of Merseyside, who later developed dementia.

'I sat next to him at a Liverpool–Southampton game and thought "goodness me",' recalls Dr Sadler. 'He was really struggling. It seemed to me we were getting more neurological illness than you'd expect.' Dr Sadler wrote to Gordon Taylor of the PFA, suggesting a study could be conducted in which former players are compared to the general public. This was in late 1993, early 1994, he estimates. 'Dismissive,' says Dr Sadler of the reply. 'I was told the PFA didn't have the sort of database which would enable us to answer that question.'

The lack of enthusiasm to examine the impact of heading and collisions still disappoints Dr Sadler. 'It's something we could have started then we'd have 20 years of a study now,' he says. He spoke to his friend Kevin Moore, the Southampton defender. They agreed it was an issue worth investigating and so, via Saints' PFA representative Iain Dowie, he tried again. 'I wrote a note for Iain to take to the next meeting, which he did, but again, it was dismissed,' said Dr Sadler. When *The Lancet* published research detailing how footballers in Finland had developed brain lesions, he thought it was worth following up on. Dr Sadler was working with the University of Southampton and confident they had the platform to kick-start a study themselves. Again, he approached the PFA, and he still has a copy of that letter. This one can be published in full.

23 July 1997

Dear Gordon,

I attach a photocopy of an article published recently in the medical journal, *The Lancet*. It demonstrates the presence of radiologically proven brain lesions in soccer players in Finland.

You may remember me writing to you on this matter a few years ago, when my thoughts had been triggered by a spate of reports on ex-footballers either prematurely dying, or developing neurological illnesses. Given the amount of times that some footballers head the ball, and the accidental trauma that they also experience, it has always seemed possible to me that some particularly vulnerable individuals may suffer a degree of brain damage.

When I wrote to you previously, asking your thoughts on whether it would be possible to attempt some preliminary study of this, you replied that the PFA did not keep a register of past players, and would thus be unable to help. You did not comment on the possibilities underlying the question.

Shortly after that correspondence, I was chatting to Kevin Moore, at that time the Saints centre-half, about this, and he was genuinely interested in the question, and how one might look to investigate it. In fact, he asked Iain Dowie, then Saints' PFA rep, to take it to the next PFA meeting, but I presume nothing further came of this.

The pace of life, and the weight of other work commitments, have meant that I have not pursued the matter further, though I have certainly not dismissed the theory.

I have been tempted to mention it to you when I have met you a couple of times in the directors' guest lounge at Blackburn, but have instead confined myself to moaning about the misfortune that always seems to accompany Southampton in their games at Blackburn!

Now with this publication, I feel that this possibility does require some investigation.

Please do not think that this is another variant of the BMA 'ban boxing' campaign. I have been a football fanatic for over 30 years, and would not countenance anything that may adversely affect the game.

It just seems to me that there is a possibility of some players suffering a degree of irreversible brain damage from their career, and that this deserves attention.

It may be that those players who are vulnerable could be identified before any significant problem is caused. I would welcome the possibility of discussing this further, and would be very interested in your thoughts.

With best wishes,

Yours sincerely,

Dr Mike Sadler

Dr Sadler says he did not receive a response. 'It's always struck me that it was a real waste,' he says in hindsight. 'I'm still a big football fan. I'm still a doctor. I watch with regret, really.' As fate would have it, Kevin Moore was diagnosed with Pick's disease – the rare condition otherwise known as frontotemporal dementia – before turning 50. Kevin died on his 55th birthday on 29 April 2013. After representing Southampton in the competition, it made him the first known victim of the Premier League era. Kevin, who dedicated a decade of service to Grimsby Town earlier in his career, was known for his excellence in the air. One of his most memorable headers was for Southampton in the 1992 Full Members' Cup Final at Wembley Stadium. 'He heads it down into the top corner,' recalls his brother Dave, pointing out that's how high Kevin could jump. 'Great spring.' Dave fears Kevin paid a heavy price for his talent, considering it 'almost inevitable' that heading contributed to his downfall. 'The thing he was most proficient at and proud of might have been what cost him everything,' adds Dave.

Dr Rowlands was still trying to make something – anything – happen as recently as 2012. That was when he received the disappointing news that the Manchester City Former Players' Association were no longer willing to participate in his research project. That was a bombshell, not least because the reason he had been pushing so hard was in the memory of Joe Mercer, the manager who presided over a gloriously golden age for City. 'I feel abandoned,' Dr Rowlands told the association. 'As will Norah.'

Researchers from Keele, Manchester and Gothenburg universities remained interested in a collaboration. For any project to work, they would need participants and so Dr Rowlands was asked for assistance. Some associations maintained that they would be happy to help, including that of Manchester United. Some wrote to say they shared his same concerns about this condition on the rise within the fraternity of former footballers and that he'd have full access to their legion of ex-players. Yet for City to withdraw their support felt like a setback – a kick in the teeth almost.

'We encountered severe difficulties throughout it all,' Dr Rowlands says. 'In getting financed. In getting players to take part. I suspected that many people did not want to go ahead with our work, lest we discovered a major problem which would affect the whole of football. We tried our best.'

Whether football's custodians can say they tried their best, that's another matter. That's on their conscience if they didn't, and Gordon Taylor insists his is clean because he did. His is a skin thicker than a rhino's, developed over four decades as chief executive of the PFA. No current Premier League player was born at the time of his appointment in 1981, giving you an idea of his longevity, and his tenure coincided with dementia in football entering the national conversation. Being the head of his union made Gordon a rich man – his extravagant seven-figure salary ensured that – and anyone who watched the 2014 Christmas special of *Celebrity University Challenge* saw his taste for the finer things in life. 'The go-to guy for footballers in trouble,' was how the show's host, Jeremy Paxman, introduced the Manchester Metropolitan University contestant who would correctly answer questions on iconic artists of the 20th century such as Sidney Nolan and L.S. Lowry. It was no surprise that he knew of the latter, given he had used £1.9m of his union's money 15 years earlier to buy Lowry's *Going To The Match*, depicting matchstick men and women making their way into Bolton Wanderers' Burnden Park. To have a knowledge of fine art is no crime, though many criticised this PFA chief for not seeing the picture being painted in front of him – the one which suggested too many of his union's members were dying with dementia for it to be a coincidence.

Now retired and having had time to reflect, there is no regret from this 77-year-old. Instead he insists the PFA were unfairly picked on, 'For all the help we've given, I'm astonished really at the criticism we've had. We helped so many people. Andy Lochhead just died and I've had a lovely message from his family for all the help the PFA gave him, for example.' He says that's one of hundreds of tokens of appreciation he's received over the years. As proof he hands me a letter sent to the PFA on 25 April 2018 from Professor Myles Gibson in which this former FA advisor expresses his dismay at the public criticism of his governance, especially in matters of head injuries. 'We've paid for respite care, home care, nursing home care, any alterations that needed doing,' Gordon adds.

A fair few families dispute that, saying they were neglected, not seen, not heard, not listened to. But Gordon is at pains to highlight the PFA's good work during his time in office. How they opposed the Football League's cap on wages. How they stopped a limit on squad sizes. How they negotiated for greater care for the health of footballers – 'the strongest contract in the sporting world, not just the football world' he says – and how they helped members get new knees or hips if they needed them. 'In the 1990s, we had Sudden Death Syndrome,' Gordon continues. 'There wasn't any testing for heart conditions, and we lobbied successfully for that.' All nice achievements, like the slice of the Premier League pie he secured for the PFA, currently worth £23m a year. But, specifically, what about dementia in football? 'I can say hand on heart we've not ignored it. It's a major issue for the whole world but at times, it's been centred on, "Well it's up to the PFA to sort it out." It's not that simple, to put it mildly.'

I ask about Dawn and Chris. That's Dawn Astle and Chris Sutton, but I don't need to mention their surnames to Gordon. He knows who I mean. They're football's most vocal and vigorous dementia campaigners who forever held him to account. They believe they're owed an apology, along with all of those other footballing families who witnessed the horrors of this disease, though Gordon doesn't feel he needs to offer one. 'Going back in time, we helped the Jeff Astle family, his wife and his daughters. Anything they asked for, they got.' The Astles dispute that, to say the least, as you'll discover in the chapter that follows. One of Gordon's final acts as chief executive was to give evidence to MPs scrutinising football's handling of brain damage in a parliamentary inquiry. As of 2021, almost 20 years on from the death of Jeff, that pioneer who never intended on pioneering, the PFA had spent a total of £1.82m supporting its members who received neurodegenerative diagnoses, helping 186 families.

Gordon is a former footballer himself and tells a story of the time he toured with Birmingham City in the United States, 'We were watching the New York Jets train. I was the smallest on the Birmingham side and they got their biggest defender to stand next to me, so it was "little and large" to illustrate the difference between their football and ours.' Different, yes, but two sports tormented by brain damage all the same. American football has adapted, with helmet-to-helmet hits now outlawed. Gordon claims he championed changes to football's concussion protocols – protocols which still fall some way short of proper protection, mind – and that he wanted a game-wide dementia fund setting up. For all these apparent accomplishments swirling around Gordon's head and spilling out his mouth, the general feeling in football has long been that he outstayed his welcome. An article in the *Mail on Sunday* on 5 April 2020, headlined 'THE LAST STAND OF FOOTBALL'S DINOSAUR', summed up that attitude towards the end of this union man's tenure. 'Dinosaur' became a familiar jibe as the PFA were accused of falling behind the times on Gordon's watch. Like how they're only now getting around to totally transferring their long list of members into a digital database, complete with neurodegenerative status.

He always was a defiant defender of his work, Gordon. He still is, clearly. Should any class-action lawsuits crop up like those seen in American football, that defence would be tested in full. Sources continuing to work nine to five at the PFA headquarters don't share the same defiance as their former leader. Though they feel the criticism has been harsh – I'll leave that to you to decide – they don't pretend the players' union was always so squeaky clean. They want to do better, and will do better, so that they don't continue to 'fall short of expectations in the eyes of the families', as one person put it. Time will tell.

In offering the FA and Premier League the opportunity to comment on the letters sent to and from the men who previously led their regimes, they pointed to the progress made of late. The heading restrictions they've recommended for training. The trial of concussion substitutes in their competitions. The partnerships with charities. The projects they've funded. That includes the FIELD study, which found footballers are more at risk of neurodegenerative disease than the regular man. It was confirmation of a link – more than two decades after these doctors' letters landed on the mahogany desks of those in charge of football.

3

# Long Live the King

*The story of the great Jeff Astle, whose death
certificate tells us he was killed by football*

'ASTLE IS THE KING' was graffitied in great big capitals on the brickwork of Primrose Bridge in Netherton, Dudley, in the heart of the Black Country, after he scored the winning goal for West Bromwich Albion in the 1968 FA Cup Final against Everton. The local authorities painted over it but that proved a waste of time. The same four words reappeared within days, and this toing and froing has continued since. It's removed. It's rewritten. Removed. Rewritten. In 1993, someone added 'PLEASE NOTE DUDLEY COUNCIL' in white paint. The council thought by installing a plaque, christening it the 'Astle Bridge', the vandals would stop. Oh how wrong they were. Visit today and you're bound to see the artwork in all its glory for yourself.

Who first wrote those words and started this delightful trend was one of football's lovely little mysteries. One rumour involved West Brom fans getting tanked up in The Round Step, a pub down the road. They watched the first final to be broadcast in colour on BBC Two then celebrated by pinching a pot of paint from the nearby workers' yard and got to writing. Yet that's not how it went down.

Today the true story can be told and there are two culprits to this tale. One is Kenny Norton, and the other is Joe Yardley, who was better known by friends as 'H' or 'Harry', his middle name. These teenage pals attended the final with 100,000 others at Wembley then caught the train home. 'We got back to Dudley Port station at about 10pm,' says Kenny, who was 18 at the time. 'We actually walked back to Netherton from there. It's about four miles but it felt like nothing because we were still so happy. We were completely sober, too, believe it or not. This wasn't the result of a day of drinking. Harry was 17 so he was too young for that anyway. We knew there was some paint in my dad's shed and that's where the idea was born. Astle was an icon. We loved him. He was someone who made our dreams come true in that West Brom shirt.'

Why they chose Primrose Bridge wasn't an accident. The local lads used to have kickabouts on Washington Street and every Wednesday, West Brom's players would pass them on their way to the Cradley Heath dog track. 'We knew they had to cross over that bridge, so that's why we chose to put the graffiti there,' continues Kenny, now 72. 'We wanted them to see it.'

When Joe died in 2014, his family had to decide where to scatter his ashes. They chose the Dudley Canal, beneath the bridge. West Brom supporters adored Jeff Astle. To them, this rugged man who scored 174 goals in 361 games over a captivating decade was and always will be known as 'The King'. He is Baggies royalty and someone who brought success to one of the Football League's founding members. He was fearless up front and, to his detriment, a commanding header of the ball.

It is now 20 years since Jeff's passing. He was diagnosed with dementia at 55 and died at 59. 'There was a black and white picture of him scoring in that FA Cup Final above the settee in the front room,' says Jeff's daughter, Dawn, welling up as she thinks back. 'After he grew forgetful, Mum asked if he knew who that man was. He said, "I don't know." She asked if he knew the team. He paused and said, "Was it Fulham?" Hearing that ripped out your heart. He just couldn't remember. My mum found an old Christmas card recently which one of us had bought for my dad to give to her. Inside he'd written "To my wife Laraine" but then at the bottom he signed it like an autograph. At the side of his signature, he'd added 78 Greenhills Road, Eastwood, which is where he lived as a boy in Nottingham. This was when the dementia was taking hold but he could still write, and you could tell it was his writing because of how shaky it was. That's why my mum kept it. She knew this might be the last one she receives from her husband.'

Jeff's disease was aggressive and his deterioration fast. 'For some it can come on gradually,' says Laraine. 'For Jeff, it came on like a juggernaut out of control. It changed him instantly. Jeff didn't realise. He had no idea, and I am glad about that.' This England international who faced Brazil at the 1970 World Cup could now only shuffle. This entertainer who would close out the comedy show *Fantasy Football League* alongside Frank Skinner and David Baddiel with a sing-song could only mumble. He would try to leave moving cars. He would try to eat inedible items. He wore adult nappies and drank from baby beakers. He was surrounded by medals and memorabilia but couldn't remember being a footballer, let alone one of the greatest of his generation. Nor could he recall the names of his three daughters, Dawn, Claire and Dorice, or any of his grandchildren, all of whom were there the day he choked to death on 19 January 2002.

That is a date permanently etched in Dawn's memory. It was a Saturday afternoon and she was celebrating her 34th birthday at her home near Burton upon Trent. Four generations of the Astle family were present for the party. Jeff sat down for dinner, and that's when it happened. He began to cough. Then it got worse. They stood him up. Still coughing. They took him outside. Still coughing. It became clear he was choking. Frantic appeals for

Jeff to spit out whatever was stuck in his throat were frivolous. His frayed mind did not have the capacity to comprehend what was happening and he was gritting his teeth together. Jeff fell to the floor, and the coughing and heaving and struggling stopped. Efforts were made to resuscitate the 59-year-old but he died, in front of Laraine and the rest of his family. Take a moment to think about that.

'I was taken over by a fog of grief,' says Dawn. 'There were dark thoughts. I could be ironing and then suddenly, from nowhere, I could see my other half Alastair and our two kids walking hand in hand to my grave. It felt real. I couldn't focus on anything other than my dad's death. I thought I was losing my mind. I was fortunate that I had the strength to say "I'm not right". My therapist said my thoughts were typical of PTSD, which is probably because of how my dad died and what we witnessed. It explained the prolonged grief. I knew it would take time to unravel and release because that's what everyone would tell me. But 20 years on, it still hasn't.'

As if this was not cruel enough, Jeff's death came a week after Laraine had lost her mother. 'We only buried her the day before Jeff died in my arms,' Laraine says. 'It jolted me. That was in January. Then one night in April I went to bed. Apart from the grief, there was nothing wrong with me physically. I woke up the next morning and from the top of my head to my toes, it was as if someone had put me in a mangle and rolled me through it. I was in pain. I couldn't move. "What's happened? Have I twisted my body in the night?" It turned out I had rheumatoid arthritis.' For those unfamiliar, it is an incurable condition in which your body's immune system becomes a saboteur as it attacks the healthy cells. Laraine continues, 'To lose my mother and Jeff so soon to one another, it jolted me. It wiped out my immune system. That's why I've been so vulnerable throughout this Covid-19 pandemic. I've lived my life wearing a mask – with a great big West Brom badge plastered on the front – and barely left my front door.'

How different it could have been, with Nottinghamshire County Cricket Club showing an interest in recruiting a young Jeff. Instead he chose football over cricket, starting his career with Notts County. Dawn had long suspected that the sport he played led to his condition. She remembers arriving at the Chapel of Rest. It was eerily silent and the coffin was directly ahead. It took time for her legs to start working. Standing over her father's body, Dawn made a vow. 'If football has done this to you,' she told him, 'I will make sure the world knows.'

Confirmation of how and why Jeff died arrived on 11 November 2002 when South Staffordshire coroner Andrew Haigh recorded a verdict of 'death by industrial disease'. In other words: death by football. The newspaper headlines outlined that clearly. 'Heading the ball killed striker' read *The Guardian*. 'Jeff Astle killed by heading ball' wrote the *Daily Telegraph*. It went worldwide, even featuring on the back page of the *Ottawa Citizen* in Ontario, Canada. 'Headers led to player's death' was the headline beneath a picture of Jeff in those famous West Brom stripes. It was the first ruling of its kind. Dr Derek Robson, the consultant neuropathologist at the Queen's Medical Centre in Nottingham, had conducted a post-mortem and told the inquest that there was 'considerable evidence of trauma to the brain similar to that of a boxer'. A further examination of Jeff's brain by neuropathologist Professor Willie Stewart later confirmed he had Chronic Traumatic Encephalopathy, making him one of the first footballers diagnosed with CTE.

As they left the coroner's court, Laraine told Dawn, Claire and Dorice that their father could not possibly be the only one. Dawn thought this would be a defining moment. She thought those in charge would want to protect the players still playing. She thought they would want to find out how many other former footballers are struggling and try to help them. She thought wrong. 'Dad's death was swept under the carpet,' she says. 'Football doesn't want to think it can be a killer. But I know it can be. How? Because it's on my dad's death certificate.'

Laraine phoned the Professional Footballers' Association after the inquest in the hope of speaking with chief executive Gordon Taylor. She says a receptionist at the players' union answered, telling her that Gordon was busy but that he would call back. He didn't. Laraine waited two weeks then tried again. And again. And again. Every time she phoned, she was told he was unavailable – in a meeting, not in the building, whatever – but that he'd call back. To this day she's never spoken with Gordon. 'Fobbed off,' Laraine says. 'I'm sure they thought, "She'll go away eventually." And I did, because I stopped calling. But we came back with a vengeance, with an army of West Brom fans behind us.'

More on that later. First, the Astles had to endure further 'fobbing'. They remember receiving two letters from the Football Association in the aftermath of Jeff's death being deemed a consequence of his career. One was sent to Jeff's widow the year after her husband's passing, advising her against pursuing damages. 'We consider any suggestion by you of a claim to be flawed, misconceived and without foundation,' stated the letter from the FA's solicitors. Laraine found it confrontational and was insulted at the suggestion that there must have been other reasons for Jeff's dementia, with no scientific research to back up that claim. She wanted to rip it to shreds and throw it away, but Dawn took it home with her instead. She still has it in her possession. The other letter was an invitation to an England international friendly in Manchester, although the FA only offered the family two tickets. 'Mum rang me,' says Dawn. 'She was distraught. Is that what her husband's life was worth? Needless to say we didn't go.'

Better news was the promise of a ten-year study into the impact of heading footballs, at a cost of £116,000 and jointly funded by the FA and PFA. The idea was they would identify and follow 50 footballers from the England youth team through their careers, collecting detailed neurological data and tracking the players' progress over the coming decade. They would be followed up at the five- and ten-year marks and compared to controls who didn't play football. For the Astles it felt like this was a real response to Jeff's demise. They were heartened by this announcement. Maybe something good would come out of their despair. However, what they hoped would be the start of something significant was instead a total failure.

It started with *Mail on Sunday* journalist Sam Peters speaking to Jim Holden, the former chief sports correspondent for the *Daily Express*. Jim had covered the initial story involving the Astles and, knowing Sam's interest in investigating concussion in sport, suggested he look into what was happening now. 'The more digging I did, the less I found,' says Sam. He chased the FA and PFA and, after overcoming a wall of silence, he discovered the study had been shelved – silently. No announcement. No press release. No phone call to the Astles, who had taken the FA and PFA's promise to research this problem in good faith and were being patient. This was 12 years after the death of Jeff.

'When Sam phoned, I thought he was going to tell me the outcome,' Laraine recalls. 'I said, "Yes! It's late! We've been wondering what was happening there." We never thought they'd try to bury it because it was so monumental for a player to die at 59 with a coroner saying what he said. If you're willing to do that for somebody who played for his country in a World Cup, what chance have others got?'

In hindsight, Dawn regrets not staying on top of the research. 'I wish I'd rang them at least once a year to ask, "How's the study going?" I didn't and I still beat myself up about that. I trusted them. My family trusted them because of the coroner's verdict. The outcome of that inquest was never challenged. Not by anybody. We assumed, incorrectly, that they were doing their duty. This wasn't about metatarsal injuries, or broken legs, or arthritis. This was something killing footballers. The study disappeared and nobody had the decency to tell us.'

Until Sam contacted them, that is. Sitting in the home where Jeff had died, he explained the situation to the unaware Astles. He told them there was no evidence to suggest a study had been completed. They were devastated, and the *Mail on Sunday* ran the story under the headline 'FOOTBALL IN THE DOCK'. This was on 23 March 2014. Sam also told the Astles about CTE. They had heard of 'boxer's brain' because that was mentioned at the coroner's inquest, but they didn't realise it had a new name or the waves it was making in America.

When Jeff died, he was initially taken to Burton District Hospital and from there sent to the Queen's Medical Centre in Nottingham. To this day the family don't know why. They assume someone at Burton recognised the name 'Jeff Astle' and, seeing that he looked closer to 99 than 59 in appearance, decided he needed sending to Nottingham for closer examination. It was there that his brain was removed – his passion for organ donation making that possible – and there it remained 12 years later. Dawn didn't know what shape it was in. Whether it was still intact. Whether it was in slides. But she wanted her father checked for CTE. She spoke with Professor Willie Stewart, who confirmed he did indeed have this trauma-induced disease. 'Willie said if he hadn't known he was looking at the brain of a 59-year-old, he'd have thought he was examining someone in his 90s,' Dawn recalls. 'Every single slice had trauma in it. All I could think was, "Was he in pain and wasn't able to tell us?" Oh God.' The tears are flowing at that thought. 'It's horrible.'

The promise of that ten-year study and its failure was the start of the Astle family's rocky relationship with the FA and PFA. Surely this was an issue that English football's governing body should want to take seriously. Surely it warranted the players' union's very existence. 'They chose the wrong family,' Laraine says, forcefully. It later transpired that some of the participants in the study left the game early and so it was truncated to five years. Gordon Taylor, the PFA's chief executive at the time, tells me the fact a pig's ear was made of this project surprised him as much as anybody. 'We were left in the dark. It wasn't as if we knew what was happening and thought, "Bugger it." It wasn't that at all.' He talks of a 'dispute' between those who were supposed to be conducting the longitudinal study (the researchers themselves dispute that) and insists the union repeatedly chased up to no avail. 'It was very strange because I thought we were all in this together,' adds Gordon, admitting no fault. Results of the research were eventually released in 2016 but the PFA went on to describe the project as 'inconclusive' and said it 'left many unanswered questions'.

The Astles responded by launching a 'Justice for Jeff' campaign. Laraine wanted an apology from the FA and a legitimate study set up – one which wouldn't silently stop like the last one. On 29 March 2014, when West Brom hosted Cardiff City, a 'Justice for Jeff' banner appeared at the Hawthorns for the first time. Supporters applauded and sang his name. BBC One's *Match of the Day* neglected to show the banner in their highlights programme later that night. But they did find time to highlight a hired plane flying over Old Trafford, calling for Manchester United manager David Moyes to leave the club. 'Moyes out' made the cut. 'Justice for Jeff' didn't.

Forcing football to take notice was one of the hurdles the Astles had to overcome. They needed to go bigger. For West Brom against Stoke City, the final game of the 2013/14 season on 11 May 2014, they had 27,000 A4 posters printed. Enough for one per person at the Hawthorns, they depicted the number nine which Jeff used to display on his back. Cradley Heath-based MSA Print refused to take money for creating the placards. The idea was supporters would hold them up in the ninth minute in honour of their greatest-ever striker. For whatever reason, West Brom didn't want these flyers being distributed on club grounds and tried to stop that from happening. Jeff's daughter Claire accused them of being 'quick to make money off my dad's memory in the club shop, but not so quick to support something which doesn't make them any profit'. Thankfully there were stewards who didn't take notice of the order. Some even stuffed a few in their pockets to sneakily hand to supporters as they entered through the turnstiles.

'I was a nervous wreck,' says Dawn. 'I was in my seat, looking up at that clock closing in on nine minutes and wondering whether anyone would hold up a flyer or if they'd be turned into paper planes. Then it's the ninth minute and oh my God, it was as if all 27,000 were lifted up at once.' It was a sea of number nines. Laraine was listening to the game on BBC Radio WM at home. 'My grandson, Joseph, was born in 2013 so he was only a baby,' she says. 'I was looking after him so Claire could go to the game and give out the cards. I could hear the supporters singing over the radio, "Are you watching, Jeremy Peace?" He was the chairman at the time.' It was in response to the Premier League club's attempt to stop the posters from making it into the Hawthorns. 'When you've got the supporters on your side, you've got one hell of an army,' Laraine adds. 'Albion fans were always like comfort blankets to us.'

Football took notice of this protest. FA chairman Greg Dyke wrote to Laraine, offering to meet. She accepted the invitation. The family were asked if they would like to be VIP guests for the Community Shield between Manchester City and

Arsenal at Wembley Stadium on 10 August, the curtain-raiser to the 2014/15 season. It risked bringing back memories of that derogatory offer of two tickets to an England friendly. 'Initially I said, "No. If they think we're going to have ten minutes before sitting back and watching a game in our posh frocks, then not a bloody chance,"' Dawn says. 'I wanted a proper meeting and, to his credit, he agreed.' In attendance were Dawn, Claire, Professor Willie Stewart and Laraine, who wanted answers and an apology. 'When I walked in, Greg held his hand out and his very first words to me were, "Nobody's bothered to listen to you, Laraine, have they?" I said, "No they haven't." He said, "Well, I'm listening now. Sit down and tell me." He was brilliant with us, and a man of his word.'

The meeting lasted for one hour and 20 minutes. Outside of Wembley, the half-and-half scarf salesmen were making their money as 71,523 fans filtered into England's national stadium. Inside, in a private room set aside for their use, the FA were finally listening. It was productive. The Astles felt heard. From there they made their way to the pre-match banquet where Greg Dyke stood up to make a speech. 'We were right next to the podium where he was stood and he introduced us to the room,' Laraine recalls. 'We didn't know how to react! His speech was shown on the televisions of all the boxes in Wembley – everybody heard it. "We owe this family a debt of gratitude," he said, and he apologised. He didn't have to do that. He'd already told us this in private.'

As half-time approached, Dawn and Claire spied a familiar face in the private box to their right-hand side. It looked like Liam Gallagher, the singer from Oasis. Their nosiness didn't go unnoticed. At half-time, they were beckoned over. It was him. 'Liam asked us if we were supporting Manchester City or Arsenal,' Dawn says. 'We told him neither! We were there because our dad was Jeff Astle, the former West Brom striker.

Liam was lovely – he asked us all about him, about his dementia, about dementia in football. He's a City fan and I told him it would affect his club, too.' It has, with Denis Law and former England centre-half Dave Watson among the high-profile players who went public with their diagnoses. 'Liam wished us the best of luck with everything, and then we tried not to stare at him too much in the second half after meeting him!' The family also bumped into Bob Wilson, the former Arsenal goalkeeper, as they were leaving Wembley. He told them Greg Dyke's speech was 'marvellous', having watched it on the television in his box.

The FA agreed to investigate why so many former footballers were being struck down by dementia. That didn't mean the Astle family were ready to put their feet up and leave it to the authorities, however. They doubled down less than a year later. On 11 April 2015, The Jeff Astle Foundation was launched. This charity's birth coincided with West Brom against Leicester City. They chose this game for two reasons. One, Jeff made his debut on 30 September 1964 for West Brom in Leicester. And two, it was a Midlands derby, and Jeff was a Midlander through and through. The club offered to help on this occasion. They told the family they would lodge a request with the Premier League to replace their regular home kit with a one-off replica strip from the 1968 FA Cup Final. Jeff achieved the feat of scoring in every round of that season's competition, so this would be a fitting tribute to 'The King'. Not a chance, the family thought. The Premier League had only allowed this to happen once before – for Manchester United in 2008 to mark the 50-year anniversary of the Munich air disaster. Yet to the Astles' amazement, permission was granted.

The sight of those red socks and white shorts and shirt brought back special memories for those old enough to recall Jeff's exploits at Wembley. No names on the back. No brands on the front. Just numbers and the crest – a strip synonymous with

Jeff. That was a special day for the Astles and after that, other families of former footballers with dementia started to approach The Jeff Astle Foundation. How many? Dawn estimates around 400, with the details of them all written down in a bundle of A4 spiral-bound notebooks. Some plied their trade in the 1960s and 1970s, like her father, but she's now hearing from families whose loved ones played in the 1980s. She sees no reason why there won't be a wave from the 1990s soon enough.

Like Laraine told her daughters outside of the coroner's court, their father couldn't be the only one. He wasn't, and Dawn became a shoulder for these suffering families. She listened to their stories. Of hardship. Of feeling forgotten. Of husbands, fathers and grandfathers dying in the most degrading of ways. She's still listening. The Jeff Astle Foundation is happy to help, Dawn says, but a significant part of their work is to pressurise the FA and PFA into doing their jobs. She wants them to be the ones fighting for the protection of players. It is too late for Jeff, but not for others.

In his post-playing career, Jeff often closed the comedy show *Fantasy Football League* with a sing-song. He would knock on the door, and Frank Skinner would answer. Sometimes he would walk in with props, like a packet of Walkers crisps when pretending to be Gary Lineker for a rendition of the Peters and Lee song 'Welcome Home'. The episode which aired on 14 April 1995 ended with Jeff walking in with a football strapped to his forehead – a nod to his reputation as someone who could score as many with his head as his feet. Good fun at the time, as Jeff proceeded to sing Kylie Minogue's 'The Loco-Motion' in front of a live audience and fellow guests Elvis Costello and Alan Hansen. A little awkward looking back now as Jeff started to show signs of deterioration just two years later.

Frank Skinner himself, now a patron of The Jeff Astle Foundation, noted this upon reflection. He was a special guest at a gala dinner at Hotel Football in Manchester on 13 May 2017, which marked what would have been the former England international's 75th birthday. During his speech, Frank recalled the time they wanted Jeff to sing 'God Save the Queen' for an episode. 'We asked him to sing the national anthem and he said, "I don't think I know it." I said, "Well you must have heard it at least five times," because he had five England caps. We laughed about it, but looking back, I do wonder if that was a sign of things to come.'

Jeff is not the only footballer whose death certificate reads 'industrial disease'. It is the same for Alan Jarvis, who died at the age of 76 in a nursing home in Mold, Flintshire, on 15 December 2019. Coroner John Gittins confirmed on 15 October 2020 that he considered Alan's job the cause, 'I am not saying playing football always causes dementia but, on the balance of probabilities in Mr Jarvis's case, his previous occupational history has been a factor in his neurogenerative functioning. It is a result of his occupation.'

Alan played throughout the 1960s and 1970s. As a Wales international, he faced England at Wembley in 1966, months after Sir Alf Ramsey's boys had been crowned world champions. Lining up against Alan that day were Sir Bobby Charlton, Jack Charlton, Nobby Stiles, Ray Wilson and Martin Peters – five men from the World Cup-winning side who were subsequently diagnosed with dementia. Alan was in his 50s when he first grew forgetful and it went downhill from there. Following his death, Alan's family donated his brain to the same neuropathologist who examined Jeff's. The damage was entirely consistent. 'There may well be more in the future as science catches up,' the coroner added at Alan's inquest.

First there was Jeff, then there was Alan. Their cases formed part of a push to have neurodegenerative disease formally recognised as an 'industrial disease'. For that to happen the

Industrial Injuries Advisory Council (IIAC) say there needs to be a 'relative risk of more than 2.0'. In other words: the risk of the disease needs to be at least doubled for those in that workplace. Former coal miners with osteoarthritis of the knee can claim financial support from the government, for example. They were exposed to hazards that others were not. This was football's argument, too. The PFA initially wrote to the IIAC in 2003 but the body refused the request two years later, saying there was not enough evidence. After the FIELD study found former footballers were three-and-a-half times more likely to die with dementia, there was arguably now proof that the 'relative risk' was 3.5. Dawn arranged a trustee meeting of The Jeff Astle Foundation in November 2019 in which she suggested they try again. 'We didn't know where to start, how it worked, what to write or who to,' says Dawn. She knew someone who might and that was Dr Judith Gates, the wife of the former Middlesbrough defender Bill Gates. On their behalf, Dr Gates submitted a paper to the IIAC citing the FIELD study. She also offered them access to an extensive archive of evidence, collated by Stephen Casper, a historian of medicine at Clarkson University in New York. It did no good, however.

There are footballers today who want for nothing and never will, thanks to their whopping wages. Those of old weren't so fortunate. The cost of caring for a former footballer in need can ruin a family. Tony Parkes is 'Mr Blackburn Rovers' – someone who played, captained, scouted and coached for the Lancashire side. He was football's greatest caretaker after keeping the manager's seat at Ewood Park warm no fewer than six times between 1986 and 2004, forever willing to serve his club. Yet following retirement, he was the one in need of care. At the age of 71 Tony moved into a home at a cost of almost £4,000 a month. It left his daughter, Natalie, lying awake at night worrying about making ends meet. She was sure football caused her father's downfall and yet it was on her to ensure Tony was cared for. Worse still, during the Covid-19 pandemic, visits meant there was a window between them. That was hard. It confused Tony. He could not understand why his daughter was on the other side of the glass, or why he could not be hugged. Tony cried, as did Natalie.

Families such as the Parkeses may not see neurodegenerative disease in sport waved through by the Industrial Injuries Advisory Council in the next decade. In a leaked letter from the IIAC, sent my way on 3 September 2021, their list of excuses for a delay was long. It said they were waiting on 'potentially important ongoing studies that may not produce results for several years'. They were prioritising other issues, including Covid-19. Resources were 'scarce', they said, and there were complications when it comes to a disease widespread among society. The letter also warned that even after the IIAC recommended Dupuytren's Contracture – otherwise known as 'miner's claw' – be added to the list of prescribed diseases in 2014, it took until late 2019 for regulations to come into force. Dementia in football, therefore, was still years from being recognised as an 'industrial disease'.

The findings of the FIELD study were not celebrated by the Astles, even if it was confirmation of their fears. 'It's like Greg Dyke said, "Nobody's listened to you, have they?" We knew there was a problem,' says Laraine. 'Too many families of players had been in touch with us after Jeff – hundreds upon hundreds. But we didn't expect it to be as bad as three-and-a-half times the risk. My first words were, "Oh the poor fools." We didn't celebrate. There was nothing to celebrate. We were proven right but you don't celebrate when lives have been lost and are still being lost. This just meant that we didn't have to justify it anymore. The word was out there now. My Jeff's brain looked like a boxer's. But he wasn't a boxer. He was a footballer and that's why we wanted answers. We wanted the truth. And we got it. By God yes, we got it. It all snowballed. A snowball that started as the size of a golf ball ended up being so big you couldn't see round it.'

Dawn never intended to become a campaigner. It was thrust upon her and the responsibility can be exhausting. She has spoken about the anguish, the funerals, the flashbacks to the day her father died, the sleepless nights thinking about this, that and the other. And yet, she has no plans to retire from the fight. She wants the authorities to step up and won't stop until they do. A sit-down with Gordon Taylor, the PFA's long-serving former chief executive whose £2m salary was the subject of much furore, at their Manchester offices some years ago ended with Dawn storming out of the room. As she stood up to leave, he said, 'That's why I've brought this file. Do you not want to have a look at how much work we've done on it?'

Adamant to the end that the PFA did its duty, 'gormless Gordon', as some of his detractors liked to refer to him, is no longer in charge of the players' union. It was announced on 27 March 2019 that he would be stepping down after 38 years at the helm, though his exit wasn't immediate. On 25 November 2020, Chris Sutton accused the 76-year-old of having 'blood on his hands' in his column for the *Daily Mail* newspaper. 'Now he says he'll be going at the end of this season,' Chris wrote. 'Why not go now? This is Taylor going out on his own terms, dictating to the very end. It is handy how between now and then, he'll take home, what, another £1m?' On 2 July 2021, some 828 days after the initial announcement, the PFA confirmed Taylor's exit. He was replaced by Maheta Molango. Dawn, along with Rachel Walden, the daughter of former Portsmouth, Gillingham and Bournemouth wing-half Rod Taylor, subsequently joined the PFA to help shape a 'dementia department'.

Though she's working with the union, that doesn't mean she's forgiven them. 'I'll never, ever forgive the PFA,' says Dawn. 'I'll never, ever forgive the FA. Because this responsibility should not have been placed on the shoulders of a family still struggling to accept what happened. I can't believe it's 20 years. It sounds morbid but that day he died, I remember everything – what I was wearing, who was where, what I was doing. Every detail. I've struggled, and I'll continue to struggle, but it's nothing compared to what my dad faced. It's been a very lonely journey for us. A frustrating one. A tearful one. But it was a journey we had to take.

'Giving up was never an option. My dad would never give up on us. Never. His death and the deaths of so many other footballers matter. There were no airs and graces about my dad. He'd speak to someone in the street the same way he'd speak to the Queen. He was always up for a laugh. One of his team-mates said, "You always knew when Jeff was in the room and to find him all you had to do was follow the sound of the laughter." I still receive messages about Jeff the footballer and they're lovely to read. The ones which mean more to me, though, are the ones about Jeff the man. How he had time for everybody. He was larger than life. That's why this void we have is just so massive.'

Jeff would be proud of his family. Dawn promised her father two decades ago she would let the world know if football could kill, and now it knows. It didn't stay in the confines of that coroner's court in Burton upon Trent. It is still discussed to this day. In this book. In newspapers. When walking through the gates named after this former goalscorer at West Brom's ground. When crossing the 'Astle Bridge' and driving by its iconic graffiti.

Around the 20-year anniversary of his death, I found an interview with Jeff in the archives. 'That final was made for me,' said the hero of West Brom's 1968 FA Cup triumph. 'I'd scored a goal in every round and on the Friday night, I think he was up there, looking down at me, saying, "Tomorrow, let's make it 1-0 and let him score the winning goal." I still believe that.

There were quite a few chances missed in the match, especially by Jimmy Husband of Everton. They all seemed to miss. I just felt the match was made for me and then this goal came in extra time. I ran to the supporters' end where we were. I could have just kept running and running, cleared over the stand and got out of the stadium. It was a dream come true. It's a thing I'll never, ever forget.'

Except he did. That black and white picture hanging in the front room faded in Jeff's mind, until finally he did not know it was himself swinging a left foot for glory at Wembley. Thanks to his family, though, his legacy will never be lost. 'His brain is now speaking for the living and I will always – always, always, always – speak for him,' says Dawn.

Long live 'The King'.

# 4

# 'Please, See That My Brain Is Given To The NFL's Brain Bank'

*The NFL, CTE, denial, damages, and an
American footballer's final request in a suicide note*

*TIME* MAGAZINE'S list of the world's 100 most influential people in 2018 was a who's who of power and fame. Donald Trump, Prince Harry and Meghan Markle were listed under 'Leaders'; Oprah Winfrey, Roger Federer and Elon Musk under 'Titans'; Jennifer Lopez and Rihanna under 'Icons'; Nicole Kidman and Hugh Jackman under 'Artists'.

Listed under 'Pioneers' was Dr Ann McKee, the accompanying picture showing her in a room draped in stainless steel and standing over a human brain, ready to dissect and discover its secrets. Some organs like to show when they're sick. Lay them side by side on a laboratory bench and an unhealthy heart can look significantly different to the healthy one, for example. The brain doesn't divulge its defects so easily. There may be some shrinkage, an early indication of impairment, but it takes looking inside to truly understand the harm inflicted upon it. This is where Dr McKee comes in. She has studied the brains of more deceased athletes than any other scientist in the world, along with military veterans. How many overall? She isn't sure. It's somewhere in the thousands, and most of them spent their lives having their heads repeatedly banged in some way, shape or form, like as a representative of the National Football League. 'She may have saved my life,' Chris Borland, the former San Francisco 49ers linebacker who retired at the age of 24, told *TIME*. 'I had dedicated my life to the game of football and realised a dream by competing in the NFL. But after just one season, I quit because I was worried about brain damage. Dr McKee's groundbreaking work on Chronic Traumatic Encephalopathy – CTE – was central to my decision.'

As someone on the front lines in these brain wars, she's encountered opposition. Not dissimilar to that which Dr Bennet Omalu faced after announcing he had found CTE in Mike Webster, the four-time Super Bowl winner who died on 24 September 2002, aged 50. The resistance to Dr Omalu's discovery of the trauma-induced disease in 'Iron Mike' was depicted in the Hollywood film *Concussion*, starring Will Smith. 'Bennet Omalu is going to war with a corporation that has 20 million people on a weekly basis craving their product,' says Dr Cyril Wecht, portrayed by Albert Brooks, in that 2015 flick. 'The NFL owns a day of the week. The same day the church used to own. Now it's theirs.' Although he gained a reputation as the global authority on CTE with this film championing his work, Dr Omalu isn't universally liked, including by those operating in similar scientific circles. He's been accused of seeking fame and fortune and fuelling misconceptions about the condition.

Dr Omalu disputes this, pointing out he was the first to discover the presence of CTE in American football and that his research withstands rigorous scrutiny by his peers. Asked about his detractors, Dr Omalu told me if he was white, maybe it would be a different story. 'My experience in the scientific community in regard to my work on and discovery of CTE epitomises the systemic exclusion and marginalisation that black physicians and scientists have historically experienced,' he says, 'whereby their hard work and ingenuity are ridiculed, dismissed and deemed inferior. Meanwhile, other physicians and scientists of Caucasian descent will claim merit for exactly the same work and creativity. I was extremely disappointed and heartbroken that this continues to happen even in the 21st century. No wonder no black person has won a Nobel Prize in Medicine. My hope is that this does not happen to my children.'

Whatever your opinion of Dr Omalu and his work, there is no denying the part he played in initiating one of the most important sports stories in history, which is still being written today by scientists including Dr McKee. It can be a competitive arena. Funding is a contentious issue – who gets it and where from. Generally, though, they're working towards the same goal and that is to understand brain damage in sport. Alzheimer's, Motor Neurone Disease and Parkinson's are all tied to the games we love to play and pay to watch. It is the scourge of CTE which has taken centre stage in American football and, unlike Dr Omalu, Dr McKee grew up a fan of the gridiron game. She's a lifelong supporter of the Green Bay Packers and she's got the Aaron Rodgers bobblehead in her office to prove it. If ever Dr McKee needs to remind herself of why she does what she does in the face of opposition, she can flick his head and watch it wobble to and fro.

Dr McKee is the director of Boston University's CTE Centre and its Brain Bank, the largest such collection in the world. Currently it is a condition which can only be diagnosed after death and so this is a treasure trove of evidence. It's an army, made up mainly of former American footballers, in whom CTE was suspected and confirmed. Whereas once they were living, breathing, tackling, sprinting, scoring human beings, now their brains are preserved in glass jars, pickled in formaldehyde. The military veterans examined knew the risks of entering combat and being jarred by blasts. Most of the athletes autopsied weren't fully aware of the perils in their pursuit of points, perhaps fooled by the false sense of security which came with their helmets. Many saw it as their duty to go big or go home. Jack Tatum, the Super Bowl winner nicknamed 'The Assassin' who died aged 61 after a heart attack, once said his 'best hits border on felonious assault'.

In 2009, Matt Birk became the first active NFL player to pledge to donate his brain once he has passed away. It's a promise which still stands. 'Lousy pun, but it's a no-brainer,' this Super Bowl winner says when asked why. 'I don't really look at it as a big deal. I'm an organ donor. Once you're dead, if my body parts can help somebody or help further the understanding of the effects of football, then I'm happy to do it.' As a centre for Minnesota Vikings and Baltimore Ravens, it was Matt's job to snap the ball back through his legs to the quarterback. A split second later, he would have to stop the oncoming opposition, defensive giants who often weigh in excess of 20 stone (about 130kg). Game after game, practice after practice, season after season; an unrelenting barrage of blows. He was a distributor of hits and a taker of them throughout his career. To his knowledge, he's suffered only three concussions in his lifetime: one in high school, one in college and one in the NFL. But it's the subconcussions which are the concern. It's the collective impact of all those whacks he took as a centre – the same particularly violent position in which Mike Webster played.

It was Chris Nowinski who convinced Matt of the merits of donating his brain. Previously a professional wrestler known as Chris Harvard, he portrayed a rich, snobby, intellectual wind-up merchant who went to Harvard University. 'Five, ten, 15 bucks, we'll own the company, you drive the trucks,' he would chant, part of his silver spoon shtick in his red shorts with a letter H printed on the backside. Chris was a genuine graduate of Harvard, too, having studied sociology. Yet he would retire from the ring a year on from his WWE debut after an accidental kick to the head from Bubba Ray Dudley on 7 June 2003.

It's no secret that wrestling is a scripted sport with the results of *Monday Night Raw* matches determined before a bell is rung. But the pain is real, and so are the repercussions of a fist, foot or folded chair to the head. That kick left the Hartford Civic Center spinning in Chris's mind. He forgot how the rest of this tag-team match against the Dudley Boyz was meant to play out. Meanwhile, a 21-stone beast proceeded to pound on him. Not his opponent's fault, of course. He wasn't to know. No one in the crowd knew that the 'Harvard boy' was no longer pretending to be hurt.

Chris's fuzziness didn't disappear. Prolonged concussion symptoms placed him in a position over which he had no control. He suffered from splitting headaches. He grew forgetful. He started to sleepwalk and almost jumped out of a window one night while dreaming he was choking. At the time it felt as if there was no way out, yet Chris was able to climb out of this concussion-induced cul-de-sac. His symptoms aren't as severe as they once were. Some still crop up from time to time, he says, with the 20-year anniversary of that kick around the corner. But Chris managed to pluck some positivity out from his plight.

In 2007, Chris co-founded the Concussion Legacy Foundation and in 2008, he helped launch the CTE Centre, the first institute in the world dedicated to the study of this condition. 'I am so thankful I put my faith in Dr McKee,' he says. 'Based on my early experiences in CTE research, I was looking to partner with a neuropathologist who was not only a brilliant scientist but whose ethics were beyond reproach. Dr McKee has shown immense courage in her willingness to fight for the truth against coordinated attempts to undermine CTE research from the sports industry.' Prior to 2005, only 45 cases of CTE had been published in the world's medical literature, almost all of them concerning boxers. Now it's part of a national conversation about how safe it is to play in the NFL. Some say it's become so noisy that it borders on scaremongering. Others counter that it is worth shouting about a disease which can leave an athlete demented.

Of the centre's first 1,000 donors, 708 were American footballers, with Chris taking on the role of chief brain recruiter. He had the nasty but necessary job of cold-calling grieving families to explain why giving to the experts in Boston could be worthwhile. Eventually, as word spread of his work, Chris started to receive calls. To this day he is still picking up the phone. It is in these conversations that he vouches for Dr McKee – for her sensitivity, for her professionalism, for her ability to provide answers. There's no one more experienced, he says, considering the countless times she's pulled on those purple surgical gloves of hers and held the very essence of a person in her hands. 'She recognises the precious gift each brain donor family makes. No one works harder than Dr McKee, and in her first 13 years of studying CTE she has published more than 100 studies and redefined everything we know about CTE and other consequence of repetitive head impacts,' Chris explains. Given his own history of traumatic brain injury, Chris lives in hope that someone, somewhere, will find a way to limit or stop him and others from losing their minds. 'As someone at high risk of CTE, I put my personal faith in her being the catalyst that will eventually lead to science developing a cure,' he tells me. 'She has proven herself to be the right person to lead this field.'

On 26 February 2014, it was announced that the Brain Bank had its first confirmed case of CTE in a footballer. 'Brain Trauma Extends to the Soccer Field' read the headline in the *New York Times*. Patrick Grange was talented. Highlights of his games show him majestically manipulating the ball and scoring for fun. He wanted to make it as a Major League Soccer star but was diagnosed with Amyotrophic Lateral Sclerosis – the degenerative disorder of the nervous system also known as Lou Gehrig's disease – at the age of 27. He died at 29 and his parents, Mike and Michele, were asked if they would donate his brain. They agreed and were told that Patrick's brain contained Stage 2 CTE, with Stage 4 being the most severe. Dr McKee told the *Times* that the damage to his frontal lobe was similar to that which she'd seen in American footballers. 'We can't say for certain that heading the ball caused his condition in this case,' she said, with Patrick having sustained concussions a few times in his footballing career, one collision costing him 17 stitches in his head. 'But it is noteworthy that he was a frequent header of the ball, and he did develop this disease.'

Scientists want to discover a way to diagnose CTE in the living rather than only the dead. They're sure they'll get there eventually, with studies showing how MRI scans could be used to detect the disease in athletes while they are still alive. The family of Dave Watson, the former England captain who won 65 caps for his country, fear he has CTE. Because he's got so much metal in him, Dave cannot have an MRI scan. CT scans he can have, though, and more than one specialist has warned the Watsons that Dave has one of the largest tears in his septum pellucidum they've ever seen. Cavum Septum Pellucidum is an abnormality which can be found in those also confirmed with CTE. 'Seeing it in Dave's brain raises the likelihood that he has CTE,' says his wife, Penny, adding it would be a 'total game-changer' to diagnose the disease *in vivo*. Why? Because it would enable scientists to explore methods which might slow down this all-too-familiar decline in ex-professional players, including Dave, via dedicated treatment. Until there is such a breakthrough, researchers will continue to rely on donors to gain a greater understanding of CTE.

Someday the brain of Matt Birk will be the subject of a search for tau, the protein which poisons the mind as it misfolds and malfunctions. It spreads to its neighbouring cells and kills them, progressively shutting down the body's most powerful organ. After being cut and sliced, Matt's brain tissue will be stained with special chemicals to make the toxic tau visible beneath a microscope. It is a painstaking process which can take months to complete. Whether the pattern specific to CTE is present in Matt's matter or not, his donation will not be in vain. None of them are. The storage room's shelves of the Brain Bank are filled with some of America's best-loved athletes; individuals who were searched for traces of the abnormal tau protein after their passing. Whether they're diagnosed with severe CTE, a mild case or as having died without a trace of the disease, the dissectors say they're always provided with answers of some kind from their donors.

Amid all this, it should be noted that the NFL have never admitted to any wrongdoing. Not when CTE was reported in Mike Webster by Dr Bennet Omalu. Not when they were sued by more than 4,500 former players who accused the corporation of concealing the dangers of concussions while glorifying and profiting from violent play. Not when it was announced on 29 August 2013 that the NFL had agreed to settle with that army of accusers for $765m, plus legal fees. A stipulation of that settlement, as outlined by former United States district judge Layn Phillips, the court-appointed mediator, was that it should not and could not be considered an admission of liability by the NFL. Some saw this agreement as a victory for the league. It sounded like a chunk of change but then to an operation that deals in billions of dollars, it wasn't so much a dent to their helmet as it was a stub to their toe. It was a manageable hit for them to take. The hope was that, by settling and not dragging this out in open court, maybe the men struggling could see their share of the deal before they were dead and buried. This was on the eve of the 2013 NFL season and big news, though it wasn't the end of the search for truth.

On 25 July 2017, the findings of a Boston University-led study were published. Dr McKee had examined the brains of 111 former NFL players and found CTE was present in 110 of them – a 99 per cent rate of positivity with most of them showing severe pathology. The study rightly highlighted its own limitations, namely that this was no random selection of NFL retirees. Most of the brains donated were from families who had seen the tell-tale signs of CTE develop in their loved ones and so, following their deaths, they sought confirmation in the only way they knew how: by donating to the Brain Bank. For widows it was a chance for closure, should they learn there was an explanation for their husband's erratic behaviour towards the end of his life.

One brain belonged to Dave Duerson, the two-time Super Bowl winner who made it his dying wish to be placed beneath a microscope. This former safety for the Chicago Bears and New York Giants played hard and fast and died at the age of 50, the victim of a self-inflicted gunshot wound to the heart. Why he didn't choose his head was indicated in a suicide note outlining a last request. 'PLEASE,' he wrote before pulling the trigger of that .38 Special, all in capitals, 'SEE THAT MY BRAIN IS GIVEN TO THE NFL'S BRAIN BANK.' This was a pool of players in whom problems were suspected. Naturally then, it was always likely that a high number would be confirmed as having CTE once inspected. This selection bias meant these results could not be considered a true representation of how rife the condition really is in American football.

Yet still, 110 out of 111 was significant. 'About 1,300 former players have died since the Boston University group began examining brains,' the *New York Times* explained to its readers, 'so even if every one of the other 1,200 players had tested negative – which even the heartiest sceptics would agree could not possibly be the case – the minimum CTE prevalence would be close to nine per cent, vastly higher than in the general population.'

It showed that this was no rare condition. It couldn't possibly be if it was present in so many former warriors of the NFL. In summary, Dr McKee outlined what all this means. 'It is no longer debatable whether or not there is a problem,' she said. 'There is a problem.'

# 5

# Now We Know – There is a Link

*Former footballers are three-and-a-half times more
likely to die with dementia, and that's a fact*

SOME 3,000 miles away from Boston University's CTE
Centre, at the Queen Elizabeth University Hospital in Glasgow,
Professor Willie Stewart would soon reach the same conclusion
as Dr Ann McKee. He too would say there is a problem, only
his would be in regard to the game played with a ball at the
feet. If its American namesake owns Sundays, then football can
claim to own Saturdays as much as any other sport. We set 6am
alarms to get from Newcastle to Norwich for a game at Carrow
Road then rush home to watch *Match of the Day* at 10.30pm.
We spend thousands of pounds per season on tickets and travel,
shirts and scarves, pies and pints. All in the name of support,
all because of our deep fascination for the game of football. We
live for Saturdays, when we can walk through those turnstiles
after a long working week. And yet research was scarce on the
repercussions of those who lace up and step over that white line
in front of us.

It is not as explicitly violent as American football, or boxing,
but then no sport encourages the use of the head quite like
football. Questions were being asked about a link to dementia,
given the chilling number of case studies, but there were few
answers. No evidence of an existential risk. No dataset to say

that footballers are in danger of developing neurodegenerative disease. Prof Stewart, principal investigator of the Glasgow Brain Injury Research Group, had a desire to fill that void. With that, the FIELD study – short for 'Football's InfluencE on Lifelong health and Dementia risk' – was launched. Funding was secured from the Football Association and Professional Footballers' Association, which was no small feat, and they got to work on 1 January 2018. Come 21 October 2019, Prof Stewart had an announcement to make. This was the day the results of 22 months of research would be revealed, rocking the game and confirming long-held suspicions.

Former footballers were three-and-a-half times more likely to die with dementia than the general population. For the first time, there was proof of a problem; facts to back up the fears. 'Landmark moment: Study confirms link between footballers and dementia' declared the back page of *The Guardian*. 'Proven: Football link to dementia' said the *Daily Telegraph*. 'Link' being the common word because that's precisely what this was. A link between something beautiful and something ugly; between football and dementia. The first time you hear a loved one forget your name is a sobering experience. This study, published in the *New England Journal of Medicine*, felt like confirmation for the families who had encountered that forgetfulness and long suspected football played a part in it. 'The truth always comes out, one way or another,' said Dawn Astle, the daughter of the legendary Jeff, who died with dementia at 59. When the coroner's inquest ruled Jeff's passing as death by football on 11 November 2002, there was scant scientific data available to back up this singular case study. FIELD was a significant shift in the other direction.

The study itself involved Prof Stewart and his group of experts in Glasgow comparing 7,676 male former professional footballers born between 1900 and 1977 to 23,028 individuals from the general population in Scotland. These substantial sample groups were matched by age, sex and degree of social deprivation, with death certificates used to determine how they died.

It turned out there were several benefits to kicking a ball around, including a reduced risk of heart disease and lung cancer. But the good news wouldn't overshadow the bad. Former footballers were five times more likely to die with Alzheimer's. Four times more likely to die with Motor Neurone Disease, the affliction which killed Middlesbrough great Willie Maddren at the age of 49. Two times more likely to die with Parkinson's, the condition which claimed the life of Liverpool legend Ray Kennedy at 70 after a 37-year fight. Three-and-a-half times more likely, overall, to develop neurodegenerative disease when compared to the man on the street.

RISK OF DEATH WITH
NEURODEGENERATIVE DISEASE IN
FORMER FOOTBALLERS
Any neurodegenerative disease – 3.53*
Alzheimer's – 5.07
Non-Alzheimer's dementias – 3.48
Motor Neurone Disease – 4.33
Parkinson's – 2.15
*times more likely compared to the general population*

It was eight months before the big reveal that Prof Stewart gained an early indication of these results. It started with PhD student Emma Russell running a rough analysis once the dataset was available and curated. They wanted an idea of what the mortality outcomes might look like in the footballers versus the controls and, lo and behold, a clear disconnect in neurodegenerative disease appeared. It took them by surprise.

'We decided to be very cautious on reporting and very, very careful over confidentiality around our analysis while Emma worked on expanding the numbers to a more complete, but still preliminary, set of data,' explains Prof Stewart.

Confident they were on to something, they met with other FIELD study members in the office of their colleague, Professor Daniel Mackay. 'I knew the findings as I had been working on the analysis for some weeks,' says Prof Stewart. 'But nobody else did. So I could watch their reactions as the numbers were slowly read out. Emma, in a monotone, flat delivery without any suggestion that anything of interest was coming at all, revealed that, actually, the risk of neurodegenerative death among our footballers was several folds higher than in the controls. At that point we're thinking, "Oh my."' Oh my, indeed. How did they react? 'The first reaction was, "This will shake things up." The second reaction was, "We need to be really careful from here on in."'

Prof Stewart knew these findings would rock football. He is not anti-sport. He is not The Man Out To Destroy Football. He grew up in Glasgow – a footballing city where you're either Celtic or Rangers, although he was clever enough to choose neither to support, thereby steering clear of a vitriolic rivalry. But for too long, injuries to knees and ankles have garnered greater attention than those inflicted on the brain. This study would go some way to changing that. First, though, they had to vet their initial findings. 'What we needed to do was take the data apart, build it back up again, take it apart, build it back up again, do it again, and again, and again,' Prof Stewart says, 'so that we were absolutely certain a point hadn't slipped somewhere, a number hadn't been missed or code written wrongly.' Checked, checked and checked again, they then presented the findings to an independent panel of their peers so they could check it for themselves, too. 'We needed to make sure that when it came out, it was as robust and secure and safe and sound as possible,' says Prof Stewart. If it wasn't, critics could poke holes in their conclusion and muddy their message – the message that playing football professionally carries a considerable risk of dementia.

It was hoped the FIELD study would act as a wake-up call, yet change was not forthcoming. Responses dripping in PR-speak were released. FA chairman Greg Clarke said, 'There are many questions that still need to be answered.' PFA chief executive Gordon Taylor offered, 'Research must continue to answer more specific questions.' FIFA said nothing, with the world governing body seemingly uninterested in using their considerable power to implement precautionary changes.

The inactivity brought to mind a 2003 tongue-in-cheek paper about the use of parachutes. Published in the *British Medical Journal*, it said that, technically, there was not enough evidence to say beyond a reasonable doubt that they save lives. The reason being there had never been a study set up to see what happens when, say, 50 people jump out of a plane without parachutes strapped to their backs. But then we can all agree, on the balance of probabilities, it's better to be wearing one if you're planning on stepping out for some fresh air at 33,000ft. 'Individuals who insist that all interventions need to be validated by a randomised controlled trial need to come down to earth with a bump,' said the study. It was a lesson in common sense and one which FIFA and football's other overlords could learn from. More research was required, sure, but many felt there was no reason why preventative action could not be taken in the meantime.

Compulsory heading restrictions could have been introduced into training, for example, or a trial set up somewhere in the world to see what the game would look like without headers. But first, football's authorities wanted confirmation of the exact 'cause' of the heightened risk. The FA invited scientists to solve that very riddle on 11 February 2021 – 479 days after former footballers were found to be three-and-a-half times more likely to die with dementia. They asked prospective applicants, 'What is the cause of the observed increased risk of death from neurodegenerative disorders in former professional footballers found in the FIELD study?' However, researchers said that was the wrong question to ask and an almost impossible one to answer.

To prove beyond a reasonable doubt that head impacts are the cause is incredibly difficult due to the typical 40-year delay between exposure and effect. You could play football professionally until 30 but be 70 by the time you're diagnosed with dementia. Your brain is such a complex network of neurons, it isn't overnight that it shuts down. The nature of the disease is that it's a gradual erosion of mental and physical function. Yet when it comes to Chronic Traumatic Encephalopathy, no drum roll is necessary when revealing the only common factor connecting football to American football to boxing to rugby. It's repetitive head trauma; the continual pounding of your brain throughout your career. On the balance of probabilities, therefore, it would be safe to presume that is the cause.

That 2003 paper on parachutes said 'only two options exist' in these predicaments, 'The first is that we accept that, under exceptional circumstances, common sense might be applied when considering the potential risks and benefits of interventions. The second is that we continue our quest for the Holy Grail of exclusively evidence-based interventions.' Campaigners felt the FIELD findings should have been enough to convince those in charge to intervene immediately, especially as it was supported by other historical studies from all over the world.

In Norway in 1989, for example, 69 players from six top-flight clubs were tested and found to have a significantly increased incidence of brain disturbances compared to the control group. 'Most likely due to neuronal damage caused by repeated minor head traumas,' it found. Two years later, another study in Norway saw 37 former internationals tested. Researchers found 81 per cent displayed mild-to-severe deficits regarding attention, concentration, memory and judgement. 'Probably the cumulative result of repeated traumas from heading the ball,' it said. In the Netherlands in 1998, a study compared 53 footballers to 27 athletes from non-contact sports, such as swimming. You've probably guessed the findings by now. The footballers fared worse than their counterparts. Looking at the players' positions, it was noted that defenders and forwards displayed the greatest impairment, indicating a correlation to the frequency with which they would head the ball. Another study in America in 2018 backed up this suggestion, saying heading was an underestimated cause of trauma.

The FIELD study and its 30,000-plus participants was the largest project to have ever looked at the risk of neurodegenerative disease in sport. Football didn't rush to react, however. Instead it felt as if thumbs were twiddled. Perhaps a few fingernails chewed, too, as the game's governors nervously contemplated the repercussions of a formal connection between football and dementia, knowing how it played out in the United States.

As of 21 October 2019, a line was drawn in the sand for those who had been sticking their heads in it. A line which could have legal implications. It was as of this day that football was told there's proof that the player on the pitch is placing himself in harm's way in comparison to the supporter in the stands. It was too late for recently retired former footballers. Their brains had taken the beatings, both concussive and subconcussive. All they could do was try not to dwell on what they now could not control. It wasn't too late for those currently playing, though, from the Premier League downwards. They could be protected.

There was a choice: err on the side of caution by making changes, or continue down the same potentially destructive path.

Ipek Tugcu is a senior associate at law firm Bolt Burdon Kemp, specialising in brain injuries. She suggests a storm is on its way, similar to the one which swept through American football. 'The truth is that we don't need to know the exact mechanism by which injuries are caused to know that the current rules, in football and rugby especially, are inadequate,' says Ipek. 'Research, coupled with the sheer number of players coming forward with early dementia, proves that the existing guidelines fail to properly protect athletes against the known risks of their job. We're now at risk of a large-scale crisis, similar to what has happened with the NFL in America, with athletes pursuing legal action for the preventable injuries they've suffered as part of their employment.' Football's authorities did respond by announcing recommendations on heading in training, saying players should not exceed ten 'high force' headers per week. These weren't compulsory, however. Clubs could ignore them without repercussions, and they were.

If robust, radical, real steps aren't taken, experts predict a rash of legal claims for football-related dementia could follow in the coming decades. Barrington Atkins, a sports disputes lawyer at law firm Stewarts, warns claimants could use a lack of action as proof of negligence, given the FIELD study told the world there was a problem. 'If clubs and organisations fail to make changes, they are exposing themselves to the risk of high-value litigation claims brought by injured players,' Barrington explains. 'The onus is on governing bodies and clubs – not the players – to have appropriate safeguarding measures in place, particularly for defenders, by limiting and monitoring the amount of times players head the ball, especially during training.'

Barrington mentions defenders because they are the ones most at risk. After digging deeper into the data, the FIELD team discovered a relationship between neurodegenerative disease among former footballers and the position they played in. Goalkeepers were the least at risk, said the study published in the journal *JAMA Neurology*. Their likelihood was statistically similar to that of the general population. Defenders were the most at risk, however. They were five times more likely to develop dementia compared to the control group.

RISK OF DEATH WITH
NEURODEGENERATIVE DISEASE BY
PLAYER POSITION
All players – 3.66*
Goalkeeper – 1.83
Defender – 4.98
Midfielder – 4.59
Forward – 2.79
*times more likely compared to the general population*

Prof Stewart knows what concussion feels like. He found out while riding his bicycle to the Queen Elizabeth University Hospital one morning before he ever embarked on his FIELD research. A car turned left and into his path, leaving pieces of a windscreen being picked out of his face. Yet this data was an enlightening discovery because it suggested football's dementia problem might have more to do with subconcussion, namely heading.

Gordon McQueen was formally diagnosed with vascular dementia at the age of 68 after showing symptoms years earlier. As a defender for Leeds United, Manchester United and Scotland, we watched him leap gloriously into the air to clear any and all danger. What we didn't see was his brain reacting to each and every impact in what is the invisible aftermath of heading a ball. Goalkeepers participate in that practice the least, defenders do it the most, and the statistics showed they were sitting on opposite ends of the neurodegenerative scale.

Prof Stewart saw this as the 'missing link', saying football should now consider whether heading was absolutely necessary. Some rolled their eyes at that suggestion, but he was only being led by the data. Newspaper match reports will refer to clashes of heads as 'sickening', though in reality, such collisions are rare. The more dependable, indeed guaranteed, source of trauma is in the heading. Further supporting this narrative, the study also looked at career length, finding those who played professionally for less than five years carried the lowest risk. Their likelihood was double that of a non-footballer. Those whose careers lasted more than 15 years faced the greatest risk as they displayed a five-fold increase. The longer your career – or the more you head the ball, you could say – the likelier you are to endure an unfortunate ending. A similar connection was found in American football in a study overseen by Dr Ann McKee. It was discovered that with each year of being a battering ram in shoulder pads comes an increased risk of CTE.

American football came from rugby, and rugby from football. It all goes back to the beautiful game. The story goes that Rugby School pupil William Webb Ellis, during a kick-about in 1823, picked up the ball and proceeded to run with it. From this disregard of the rules, a new sport was born, which is why the Rugby World Cup's trophy is named after young William today, his name engraved into its 24-carat gold plate. Whether true or merely a myth, who knows. One originated from the other, so says folklore, and they often cross over in Prof Stewart's line of work, too.

Families fearful that their loved one's devotion to their sport cost them everything have turned to him for confirmation. 'My first priority to them is not research,' he says of brain donations. 'It's giving them a diagnosis.' Over the years, he and colleagues have noticed a trend. When examining the brains of footballers and rugby players who died with dementia, three in every four displayed CTE pathology. Its pattern is so distinctive that scientists can see the difference between this and, say, the presence of Alzheimer's. CTE isn't always the sole cause of their demise; sometimes there is a 'normal' dementia pathology to go with it. But three in four is enough to indicate that these players' livelihoods *do* leave lasting marks on the brain.

Prof Stewart was trusted with the brain of Nobby Stiles, the England midfielder and 1966 World Cup winner who developed dementia and died on 30 October 2020, aged 78. After receiving a donation, he needs to ask a few awkward questions of the family. Did your father drink? Did he do drugs? Did he get into fights? Dementia is a complicated disorder which can be influenced by the lifestyle that particular person led. Occasionally Prof Stewart will be told about how they may have tried cannabis once or twice back in the 1960s, but that isn't what he means. He means methamphetamine, cocaine, opioids – drugs associated with cognitive decline. The answer he hears from families, time and again, is no, no and no. He wasn't an alcoholic. He wasn't a drug addict. He wasn't aggressive or some sort of Saturday night bar brawler. 'These are athletes,' he reminds me. 'A lot of them were clean-living and healthy.'

Prof Stewart confirmed CTE in Nobby. Its presence was severe and, in ruling out other factors, including the fact there was no history of him sustaining a brain injury, he proposed the risk came from heading the ball. Nobby's son, John, felt 'angered and vindicated' by the news. 'When Willie told us, it confirmed everything we'd been thinking in our own minds,' he tells me. 'I was enraged that nothing was ever done to help him.' A former professional footballer himself, John became a vigorous campaigner on behalf of today's players. His passion is not entirely embraced, even by the clubs he once represented.

One visit to the training ground of Doncaster Rovers to hand out pamphlets to players warning them about the dangers of heading the ball was in vain. John played for Rovers between 1989 and 1992 but was told he wasn't welcome and to leave.

There are those who consider this a problem of the past. They pin it on the prehistoric concussion protocols, when magic sponges were a feature of any medical man's pack. They blame it on those old leather balls. Those naysayers frustrate the people in pursuit of facts. 'What will happen in 30 years?' Prof Stewart asks hypothetically. 'We could repeat the study. We could call it "FIELD 2.0". God forbid we find the same thing. What then?'

By then, it is expected the old excuses will have been replaced by ones more fitting for 2050. Perhaps players are having their saliva tested for concussion pitchside. Maybe the balls are made from brand new materials, nothing like those old synthetic Nike lumps of 2020. It will be a copy and paste of deflection and denial. 'They'll say, "Football in 2050 is nothing like it was in 2020." People can then bury their heads in the sand and carry on for another 30 years.' To believe that all is fine because technology is as advanced as it's ever been is a failure of intelligence. Studies will continue to be conducted, all with the aim of gaining a greater picture of football's dementia problem and what could be done to reduce the risk. Thanks to the FIELD study's findings we know one thing at least – there is a link.

# 6

# Football Without Heading

*'If God had wanted us to play football in the clouds,*
*he'd have put grass up there'*

'FOOTBALL WITHOUT HEADING' read the headlines on 9 February 1938, the day it was announced that Arsenal would be engaging in an unusual experiment. 'Recently it has been argued in some quarters that there is too much heading in first-class football today,' readers were told. As a result, Arsenal's players, preparing for their FA Cup fifth-round tie with Preston North End, would play a portion of their practice match without heading the ball. Goodbye aerial duels. Hello football on the floor. Arsenal manager George Allison, who would win them the First Division title later that season, wasn't the biggest fan of what he witnessed, however. 'Admirable for practice purposes,' he said. 'It teaches players, and especially youngsters, to "kill" the ball, work it and manoeuvre with it. For league and cup tie games it is not a practical proposition. I cannot see "no heading" football being tolerated by Football League clubs.'

Arsenal lost 1-0 to Preston, the eventual winners of the 1938 FA Cup. Funnily enough, it was the visitors' preference for playing on the ground that secured them victory in front of 72,121 fans on a blustery day at Highbury. This was reflected in the Sunday newspapers' match reports. 'Preston were better able to overcome the conditions,' read one in *Reynolds News*.

'When they kept Arsenal out in the first half against a breeze that sent programmes – and not a few hats – swirling away in the direction of Highbury Barn, they showed us some really clever football. They kept the ball low, whereas Arsenal too often ballooned it badly.'

Arsenal's no-heading warm-up match was conducted out of curiosity and for stylistic purposes rather than with players' wellbeing in mind. 'A bit of fun,' as the manager described it. Because who could imagine football without heading? This is the game where that strapping lad at the back uses the flat of his forehead to propel the ball away from his box. The game where players tussle at corners and long throw-ins and a bullet header brings a stadium to its feet. The game where Andy Carroll generates more than £50m in transfer fees, largely thanks to his aerial ability.

Woodpeckers have fascinated scientists for decades for the way they're designed to withstand trauma. As explained in the prologue of *League of Denial* – the book about American football's dismissive attitude towards brain damage – they can peck at a tree trunk 12,000 times a day and suffer no consequences. We aren't so fortunate. We don't have shock absorbers installed to protect our breakable brains. We aren't built for banging our heads like the robust woodpecker and the concern of heading's impact is nothing new. Even Dr Alan Bass, the doctor to the England 1966 team, feared it isn't so innocuous. 'Being hit on the head by a fast-moving soggy ball can't be all that different to the effect of a punch,' he told the *Sunday Times* on 3 November 1974.

Over time, the link between football and dementia went from being feared to researched to recognised officially. That came in the form of the FIELD study, as detailed in the previous chapter. Yet even when those findings were released on 21 October 2019, experts resisted calling for a trial of football without heading. They had their suspicions of the cause. Heading the ball is the most obvious source of subconcussive blows, inflicted day after day and season after season, so it's probably that. But 'probably' wasn't going to cut it. They needed proof. They could say there was a connection but that's all. There was no evidence to say heading is the fatal reason why former footballers are three-and-a-half times more likely to develop such problems. Certainly not enough to convince football's stubborn custodians that they should consider changes which, if eventually implemented, would shake the world's most popular sport to its core. So Professor Willie Stewart and his team at the University of Glasgow went back to work.

On 2 August 2021, they had the necessary evidence which would enable them to suggest heading the ball *is* the trigger, finding football's dementia problem was linked to field position. Goalkeepers, who hardly ever head the ball, were least likely to develop neurodegenerative disease. Defenders, who practise it aplenty, were most likely. Five times more likely, to be precise.

Suddenly there was a legitimate reason to propose a trial, so Prof Stewart pushed the big red button he'd been reluctant to press. He asked a simple yet significant question, 'Is heading a football absolutely necessary to the game of football? Or can some other form of the game be considered?' Prof Stewart wasn't demanding football save itself from further damage. He wasn't insisting on an immediate ban on heading. Instead he was simply asking the authorities to consider its necessity. What would it look like? Would it be boring? Would it be better? How would goal kicks be brought down? How would a wall react to a head-height free kick? Crucially, would it look like football? Only through a trial would we know whether this is feasible or fanciful.

Mark Bright says if he could go back and do it all again, he wouldn't head the ball as much as he did in training. A player for Port Vale, Leicester City, Crystal Palace, Sheffield

Wednesday and more, Mark crossed paths with thousands of players; enough to fill a phonebook. Only two men ever refused to practise heading. One was Gary Lineker, who says he felt it was 'unwise' to take such a shock to his head unless it was for the benefit of scoring on a Saturday. He insisted it was something he could do instinctively in the moment, and he was right. Of Gary's 48 goals for England, 15 were headers. His refusal never hindered him in matches.

The other man who would never head the ball in training was Bob Newton. Why? 'I didn't think it was good for me,' Bob says. 'Would you ask me to go bang my head against the dressing room wall, two hours at a time, three days a week? Absolutely not. You'd think I was barmy if I did that, so that's what I'd tell my coaches. I'm my own man.' And a man ahead of his time. Bob is a chatty character who adores football and that incomparable feeling that performing in front of fans gave him. He operated in the lower reaches of the Football League and goals were his game, scoring them while centre-halves hacked away. His first professional contract came with Huddersfield Town in 1973. Even then, as a 17-year-old whippersnapper excitedly embarking on a career in football, he didn't want to head the ball. Ian Greaves was Bob's manager and, to his credit, he did not try to change this teenager's mind. 'He was totally supportive,' says Bob of his old boss, 'when other coaches might not have been so kind towards a kid.'

There was a time when Bob plied his trade as a 'soccer' player in the United States, facing Johan Cruyff, Franz Beckenbauer, Gerd Müller, Johan Neeskens and Teófilo Cubillas. Not a bad five-a-side team, that. Now 65 years old, Bob still loves a kick-about with mates in his native Chesterfield (no heading, of course). It was for his hometown club that he shared a changing room with Ernie Moss after playing together at Port Vale. Ernie died on 11 July 2021 at the age of 71, years after being diagnosed with Pick's disease, a rare form of dementia. 'They used to practise knocking balls towards the far post and heading it down, with Ernie coming in and finishing it. Then they'd say, "Right, switch around," and I'd say, "Nah, I'm not doing that." I did gain a reputation. "Everybody else is doing it. Why aren't you?" But I just didn't see it as being a good thing to be heading ball after ball at 100mph. It wasn't for me.'

This didn't mean Bob was a shrinking violet on a Saturday. If a cross came in, he turned into a steam train not to be beaten. 'Boots on, boom, I was ready. When I played football, I gave 100 per cent because I wanted to give those supporters who had worked all week and paid to see us some pleasure. I can't think of another job where you can go out and make people that happy just by scoring a goal. You're sharing a passion for 90 minutes and they were my inspiration. I loved playing for Hartlepool United, and I loved playing for Port Vale, but representing my hometown Chesterfield, in front of my mates who I went to school with, was like playing for England to me. I'd head the ball come crunch time, but never during the week. I played with players who were world-beaters in training. But on a Saturday they couldn't beat an egg. You can have that dedication to bettering your game in training – your first touch, your skills, I'd work on that, no problem, because that's a different ball game – but I never saw heading as a part of that. I didn't think it would have any effect on my game, but I did think it would have an effect on me, so I didn't do it.'

It is curious why more footballers don't refuse in the way that Gary Lineker and Bob Newton did. In games they have no choice – not while the rules are what they are. In training, though, they do. Maybe it's the pressure of their peers, of their coaches, of their clubs with whom they're contracted. Terry Butcher did as he was told and he has made up his mind, urging football to distance itself from heading altogether. 'It is something that we can do without,' says the ex-England skipper whose white shirt was stained red by an infamous head wound on 6 September 1989. It was in a World Cup qualifier against Sweden and he played on, despite bleeding profusely. Now he is appreciative of the potentially 'catastrophic' consequences of football. When someone of his stature is willing to speak as boldly as this, it's worth listening – or trialling.

Over to you, then, guardians of the game. As football's world governing body, FIFA's old slogan was 'For the Good of the Game'. Then on 31 May 2007, they announced a shiny new one. 'For the Game. For the World' would now feature on any letterheads coming out of the FIFA headquarters in Zurich, Switzerland. This switch was meant to symbolise their determination to 'develop the game' and 'build a better future'. Looking at how to limit the number of former footballers developing dementia fits that criteria.

FIFA love a trial, too. With the game's lawmakers, the International Football Association Board, one of their most recent test runs involved offsides. 'We will test a potential change to the offside law,' announced FIFA president Gianni Infantino on 5 March 2021, 'which has only changed twice in 135 years of IFAB.' It was changed in 1925, following trials, and in 1990, following trials. Now, they were trialling Arsène Wenger's latest idea to give advantage to the attackers in offside situations. 'Such a change will be tested and if it is positive we might go ahead,' the head of FIFA continued. 'If it's negative we stand back. Our aim as IFAB is always to see if we can make football more attractive – without changing the nature, obviously, of football.'

They don't want to render the game unrecognisable and that's understandable. But then the counter-argument is nobody has ever lost their life because of a close offside call. Or from a goalkeeper picking up a back pass. Or from a striker sneakily using his hand to score a goal. Yet the Laws of the Game were altered for those situations. Professor Willie Stewart's point was a trial of football without heading could literally be the difference between life and death and that it was worth consideration. If it turns out the spectacle suffers and it's not a feasible option going forward, fine, at least we know. Then the game could continue as is, perhaps with protocols in place in training instead. But until an official trial is organised, we'll never know.

Peter Crouch scored 53 headed goals in the Premier League – the most in the competition's history. He's proud of his record, although with that pride comes concern. 'I'm not naive enough to think that I am not at risk,' says the former England striker. 'There was a point in my career, when I was playing week in, week out, that I was heading a ball more than anyone in Europe's four main leagues by some considerable distance.' Clubs hire analysts to compile data such as this and pass the information on to the players. It's a way of motivating them to move to the top of the list and stay there. Peter originally dreamed of being the next Paul Gascoigne but as a 6ft-plus 15-year-old prospect, he was told to focus on using his height instead. So he practised putting that to use. A lot. 'There were times I can remember when I was literally seeing stars after sessions from using my head so much,' adds the only Premier League player to have scored a half-century of headers.

Peter might have managed a few more had Sir Clive Woodward, in his role as Southampton's performance director, followed through with his idea of having the striker lifted up for corners like a second row in rugby. Nevertheless, 53 was a nice number; more than Alan Shearer's 46, Dion Dublin's 45 and Les Ferdinand's 40. Now retired and in his early 40s, Peter is interested in any medical examinations which could tell him whether his heading prowess left a permanent mark. Whether he should be worried. Whether he is looking like one of the lucky ones.

Peter's first column for the *Daily Mail* was published on 18 November 2017, six days after Alan Shearer's BBC documentary *Dementia, Football and Me*. In that programme, viewers were shown how a brain inside the skull can wobble like jelly on a plate upon impact. Seeing that disturbed Peter and made him want to be tested for Chronic Traumatic Encephalopathy once it's detectable in the living, although it didn't stop him from doing his day job. Two days after using his debut column in the *Mail* to voice his concerns, he was in a Stoke City shirt, throwing himself at crosses against Brighton & Hove Albion. In a way, someone like Peter should want heading banned – that way his Premier League record of 53 headed goals would never be beaten. Yet he fears such a move would 'alter the sport completely'. Because of that, he says he cannot advocate a complete ban. But he says football cannot ignore the fact there is a problem here.

What's your favourite headed goal of all time? No offence to Crouchy, but mine was Lionel Messi's against Manchester United in the 2009 Champions League Final. The way he leaped in the air like a salmon out of water. The way he angled his body. Not bad for someone standing all of 5ft 7in tall. You might nominate Robin van Persie's leaping header against Spain at the 2014 World Cup, Steven Gerrard's comeback kick-starter in the 2005 Champions League Final, Javier Hernández heading backwards against Stoke City in the Premier League in 2010 or Marco van Basten stooping to head beyond Real Madrid in 1989, if you're old enough to remember that. Or any one of Cristiano Ronaldo's almost superhuman springs. The Portuguese superstar became the greatest goalscorer in the history of men's international football on 1 September 2021 with two goals against the Republic of Ireland in a World Cup qualifier. Both of them headers, they took him to 111. Of those, 25 were scored with his left foot, 58 with his right, and 28 with his head. It's a weapon of his, as Ireland discovered to their cost on a historic night in the Algarve. If heading was outlawed, those majestic moments would be lost.

Yet maybe there is a way they can be saved. Maybe it doesn't have to be that all heading is banned. Maybe they trial matches where it is only allowed inside of the penalty area. Not since 26 April 2003, when Alan Smith netted against Blackburn Rovers for Leeds United, has a player used his noggin to score from outside in the Premier League. The statistics say the majority of heading takes place around the centre of the pitch. That's where most of the damage is done on matchdays, such as when a goal kick is thundered back in the opposite direction. For every ten headers, it's said that only one of those occurs in the opposition box. If the other nine were taken away, would they be missed? Only one way to find out. A trial, where heading the ball outside of the box is removed but the prospect of a player heading home inside is retained.

There is an argument that the modern-day game is already much more focused on keeping the ball on the carpet. There was a time when English football was obsessed with route one and its biggest cheerleader was Charles Hughes, the Football Association's former director of coaching. He was besotted with long balls, to the extent that he wrote a book about why it's the best way forward. 'The strategy of direct play,' insists the introduction of *The Winning Formula*, 'is far preferable to that of possession football. The facts are irrefutable and the evidence overwhelming.' According to this influential FA official, the game was about getting into the 'Position Of Maximum Opportunity', otherwise known as 'POMO', and doing that as directly as possible. 'Patient possession football does not produce the goals that win matches,' he declared. This book would become the FA's principal coaching manual following its publication in 1990.

Not everyone in England agreed with this attitude. 'I want to establish without any shadow of a doubt that Charles Hughes is totally wrong in his approach to football,' said Brian Clough, blunt as ever. 'He believes that footballs should come down with icicles on them.' The English game has moved on from the one-dimensional manuscript that was *The Winning Formula*. Today there's tiki-taka, gegenpressing, goalkeepers playing out from the back and false nines getting between the lines. Opta's passing statistics go back to 2003/04 and they say the typical Premier League game averaged 781 passes that season. It's gradually increased since. In 2010/11 it went above 800 for the first time. In 2017/18 it went above 900. In 2020/21 it was 945, its highest to date. With managers fixated on seeing football played on the floor more than ever before, it's creeping closer to that 1,000 mark. Some of the game's biggest names have been against lumping it long for the sake of it. Think Pep Guardiola. Think Arsène Wenger. Think Johan Cruyff. Think Brian Clough, whose Nottingham Forest side won the 1979 European Cup courtesy of a back-post header by Trevor Francis. Even he wasn't fond. 'If God had wanted us to play football in the clouds,' the former Forest manager quipped in another iconic quote, 'he'd have put grass up there.'

The modern era's emphasis on passing doesn't mean heading has been eradicated, however. Barnsley against Birmingham City in the Championship on 6 March 2021 went viral because of a 45-second passage of play in which there were 19 headers. When such a sequence crops up in a Premier League game – and the top level isn't immune to a spot of head tennis – it'll prompt sarcastic comments. 'Best league in the world' and all that. Three months after signing for Chelsea from Paris Saint-Germain, Thiago Silva told reporters he was feeling the effects of English football. 'I've had a terrible headache,' revealed the 36-year-old Brazilian centre-back, 'because there are non-stop aerial duels and a very high pace of play.' Internationally, too, heading is still very much there. The Euro 2020 meeting between England and Germany at Wembley saw more headers than the 1966 World Cup Final between the same nations all those years ago.

The truth is, in a game, you aren't guaranteed to head the ball. In training, you are. That's where the majority of heading is conducted. In dedicated drills. In practice matches. In friendly warm-ups on the teqball table, which has grown in popularity at training grounds (essentially a football version of table tennis; West Ham United have even installed one outside of their press conference room at their Rush Green base). Former Premier League winner-turned-pundit Chris Sutton estimates he headed the ball 100 times a week, 40 weeks a year, for 18 years. That's 72,000 times his brain was left jiggling inside of his skull. It's numbers such as that which feed scientists' fears that football's dementia problem is primarily to do with heading the ball – more so than the three times Chris was concussed in his career. One popular training drill involved players lining up on the edge of the box. The ball would be booted from the opponents' half and the aim of the game was to head it back over the halfway line. If you didn't, it wasn't a good enough clearance.

The *Football Association Book for Boys*, published by English football's governing body in 1949, was a guide for wannabe footballers. It included a selection of articles written by some of the game's greats. Preston North End winger Sir Tom Finney penned a piece on the art of mastering the ball. Stan Mortensen of Blackpool outlined what it took to become a skilled inside-forward. In an effort at making some of its lessons easily digestible for the younger readers, the FA also created their own cartoon strip. It starred Mr Wrinkle and Dan. One was an old-school coach, the other a schoolboy. Mr Wrinkle's first lesson in the *Book for Boys* was in the importance of practising heading. The storyline started with Dan feeling embarrassed after missing the ball entirely when leaping for a cross, only for the opposition to charge up the other end and score.

Mr Wrinkle had some advice for Dan at full time. Don't close your eyes and hope for the best, says this moustached mentor in a flat cap, sheepskin coat and with pipe in mouth – keep them open until you get a headful of leather. Dan takes this on board. He spends the rest of the week heading at a target on a brick wall, perfecting his technique. Lo and behold, when the same chance comes his way the following week, he heads home the winner. 'With practice,' Mr Wrinkle says in summary, 'you can flick the ball wherever you want.'

This cartoon, headlined 'USE YOUR HEAD', is very much a product of its time, as is the column written by Joe Mercer, the ex-England international encouraging youngsters to practise pounding a ball against a brick wall. 'I remember when we were visiting Germany about 1936,' wrote the man who would go on to develop dementia, 'we saw a player there in a back yard. He went on heading the ball up, and up, and up, for long stretches to perfect his heading. How many times do you think you could head a ball to a wall and prevent it from touching the ground? This German looked as though he could go on heading until his neck broke.' An Arsenal defender at the time, he described this as 'the only way to perfect your control'. Joe Davis didn't win the World Snooker Championship by only playing in public events. Nor did Sam Snead win the PGA Championship by rocking up on the day with a bag of clubs. They practised, practised, then practised some more in private. This advice about training individually is underlined in another section of the *Book for Boys* which says readers should 'practise heading a ball continuously yourself', because that's what professional players do.

You won't find the FA offering this advice now. On 24 February 2020, fearful of the damage it was doing, children of primary school age were banned from using their heads in training. English football has taken tentative steps to try to contain this at professional level, too. On 28 July 2021 it was announced that players should limit how many 'high force' headers they complete in training – 'high force' being those that come from corners, crosses, free kicks or long passes of more than 35 metres. Guidelines restricted players to ten of these per week. How this magic number was selected was a little mysterious, as was the reason why 'low force' headers were fine to remain unlimited. The primary problem with these recommendations, though, was that they were just that: recommendations. It was guidance which did not need to be followed.

Less than two months after the announcement of these heading restrictions, Nuno Espírito Santo of Tottenham Hotspur became the first Premier League manager to admit that they were ignoring the guidelines. He'd spent his press conference complaining about how his side were conceding from set pieces, so I asked how they improve at them if they're limited in their practice. 'Good question,' he answered. 'That's why we have training sessions without nobody seeing us.' True. These guidelines were not being policed by the Premier League, or the FA, or anyone with authority. Instead players were expected to count how many headers they conducted per week, and coaches were supposed to shape sessions around this new guidance. Critics described this as impractical. Picture an academy prospect training with the first team. He pulls out of a cross and tells his coach he couldn't head the ball because he's had his ten for the week. It wouldn't happen.

'I'm concerned with the situation of dementia and what heading the ball can cause,' continued Nuno, a former goalkeeper. 'It's a big concern for us but it's part of the game. Honestly, I will not lie to you. I don't count how many times our players head the ball. Maybe I will get myself in trouble for this. But football is jumping, heading; it's part of the game.' Tottenham were not alone in ignoring the limits. After Nuno's revelation, I asked other clubs how they were complying with the new directives and not a single one would comment. It was a wall of silence.

Following a parliamentary inquiry into brain injury, MPs said sport had been allowed to 'mark its own homework'. Telling clubs to enforce restrictions which weren't even mandatory felt an extension of that conclusion, like trusting vampires to guard the blood bank as Chris Sutton put it to me. Guidelines are nice. Whether they're followed is another matter, however. The opening game of the 2021/22 Premier League season saw Brentford host Arsenal under the lights of the Brentford Community Stadium. With colleagues, I watched a heading drill in the warm-up. Coaches were throwing balls high up in the air for defenders to drive forward and head them clear. Thump. Thump. Thump. Only ten a week were allowed, although the clubs could handily claim these headers were not of a 'high force' nature.

Naturally if heading the ball was removed from the games themselves, it wouldn't need practising in training or warm-ups. Before banning primary school children, the FA researched how often those age groups were heading in matches. The number wasn't substantial at all and so they decided there was no harm in its removal from their training sessions. Maybe from their matches soon enough, too. For the professional game it isn't so straightforward.

You might have played 'headers and volleys' on the playground. You might have scored the odd goal using your head. You might have celebrated a header scored by the striker of your club. Maybe someday all of this will be outlawed. Maybe not. There will be opposition because this isn't some small tweak. Heading goes back to the beginning of the game. The first World Cup Final on 30 July 1930 saw a one-armed man secure Uruguay a 4-2 victory against Argentina using, you guessed it, his noggin. Héctor Castro had lost his right arm in an accident aged 13. The story goes that the handsome Héctor would use his stump when leaping for headers to whack anyone who dared try to get in his way. Known as 'El Divino Manco', meaning 'The One-Armed God', he confirmed Uruguay as the inaugural world champions with his head.

Could football really get rid of something so historic? Researchers say playing the game reduces your risk of heart disease and lung cancer. We're yet to see a study state heading the ball is good for you. It sounds obvious to say that the delicate brain is not designed to be bashed, but then athletes have the freedom to put themselves in harm's way if they wish. If boxers are permitted to punch, and American footballers allowed to tackle, why should football not let its players head to their heart's content? It's a valid argument. So long as the weight of evidence suggests there is a potentially deadly price to pay for heading the ball, however, this debate will rumble on. Not in my lifetime, or yours probably, but perhaps one day this will all come to a head.

# 7

# The Spennymoor Test Run

*Just a spot of fun, a charity kick-about, or a*
*potential glimpse into the game's future?*

THERE WERE two minutes and 56 seconds on the clock at
Spennymoor Town's Brewery Field when the game's first foul
was awarded. The culprit was Mark Tinkler and his crime was
heading the ball. Cue mocking cheers from the 390 supporters
in the stands. The former Leeds United midfielder and now
Middlesbrough academy coach had clearly forgotten the rules
of this experiment: no heading outside of the box in the first
half, and no heading whatsoever in the second half. Put it
down to instinct, perhaps. The ball was lumped long and flying
towards Mark. Naturally, then, he headed it back in the opposite
direction. 'I was only testing the referee,' claimed the 46-year-old
as his team-mates teased him for his mistake so soon into this
contest. 'I swear.' Yeah, right.

It was on 26 September 2021 when this footballing first
was held: an adult 11-a-side match with heading restrictions in
place. This modest home of a National League North side in
north-eastern England was not the most obvious choice of venue
for the start of a revolution. But then a sunny Sunday afternoon
in Spennymoor seemed as nice a place as any to test an idea.
With the game's governing bodies in no hurry to set up a trial of
football without heading, campaigners took it upon themselves

to conduct one. Organised by the brain health charity Head for Change, in association with the Solan Connor Fawcett Family Cancer Trust, this was their way of showing how easily such an event could be set up. If we can do it, so can you, essentially.

It was Spennymoor, representing Team Solan, versus Middlesbrough, on behalf of Head for Change. The teams would be made up of former professional footballers – such as Steve Howey, the former Newcastle United, Manchester City and England defender, and Tommy Miller, formerly of Hartlepool United, Ipswich Town and Sunderland – and me. An invitation landed in my inbox a few weeks before the big day. It was an offer to snub my seat in the stands – which was where colleagues from the BBC, ITV, Sky Sports, *The Times*, the *Daily Telegraph*, even German broadcasting giant ARD and more would be sitting – and bring my boots along instead.

That fear of sticking out like a sore thumb as an amateur going up against former footballers, men who were paid to play, needed swallowing. Ian Wooldridge was one of the *Daily Mail*'s finest reporters. He flew with the Red Arrows. He drove a dog sled across Alaska. He ran from the bulls at Pamplona. He would throw himself into the thick of it, feeling that some opportunities should not be turned down. It wasn't as death-defying as braving the Cresta Run or steering a 26 ton, 65ft, £400,000 yacht through choppy Indian Ocean waters – two more assignments for 'Woolers', who couldn't even swim – but this felt like one of those. It was an invitation worth accepting for an up close and personal view of this unique clash.

This charity match was to be the first fixture of its kind in football. It was an experiment which would enable us to see what the world's most popular sport would look like if heading restrictions were ever implemented. It was a starting point for a conversation about whether the spectacle could survive. It wasn't entirely embraced. Social media asked, 'What next? Helmets?'

but at least it got the debate going. As a tribute we would wear the names of former footballers on our backs. I was placed on the Middlesbrough team and so represented Alan Peacock, the Boro legend who developed dementia. This former England international's career ended prematurely at the age of 30. At the time he was devastated. Later he would come to consider it a blessing, admitting, 'Although my career was sadly and devastatingly cut short due to injury, I actually feel lucky. Perhaps if I had carried on playing, I might have been affected at a much younger age.'

The asking price for this potential glimpse into the future was £5 for adults and £1 for children. Supporters of age could pick up a pint of Moors Lager for £2.20, find a seat and watch us warm up, no heading practice necessary. At 2.35pm, it's 25 minutes until kick-off and towering over me on the sidelines of Spennymoor's Brewery Field is Gary Pallister. The former Manchester United, Middlesbrough and England centre-back isn't playing. He's here as a fan. Curiosity brought him here because he wants to see first-hand whether football without heading can work. As a player Gary was blighted by migraines. Four or five a season, he estimates, and they lasted the entirety of his career. As we speak this 6ft 4in colossus starts to list the symptoms, 'Blindness, loss of speech, shocking headaches.' They were debilitating and would last for two days at a time. Two days of sitting in a darkened room. Two days of throwing up. Two days of misery. 'But once I finished playing football, once I stopped heading the ball, my migraines started to subside,' he says.

It was alongside Steve Bruce, a man with the unmistakable nose of a centre-half and the bedrock on which Sir Alex Ferguson built his first era of success at Old Trafford, that Gary would practise heading daily. He says, 'I used to think then, "Is this in any way linked with football?" You had suspicions but no medical evidence and nobody saying you needed protecting. Heading is a big part of football. You're forever practising it. Now I think about the amount of times I headed the ball in training, the concussions I had, and wonder what the consequences of all that were.'

This four-time Premier League winner took plenty of whacks as a player. On 28 January 1990, for example, he was sick on the coach journey home to Manchester after a particularly severe clash of heads during an FA Cup meeting with Hereford United. But that isn't the main reason why this man mountain believes he was tormented by migraines from age 16 to 36, when he retired. The trigger, he reckons, was heading the ball. It is why he wants it removed from the children's game entirely rather than only in training. Why he wants adults properly educated on the risks. Why he found this match in Spennymoor so intriguing. There will forever be a risk of harm when taking to the field – our entire worlds cannot be bubble-wrapped – but to not explore ways of evolving football would be foolish.

So here we are. At 2.45pm, we're in the Middlesbrough changing room and Craig Hignett's boots are deteriorating. He snaps off a stud. Then another. And another. Players laugh at his predicament as they're thrown on the floor, one by one. To any Boro fans who saw this midfielder in his pomp these might be considered fun pieces of memorabilia for the bookshelf. But to the man himself, it's an inconvenience he doesn't need 15 minutes before the start of this match. When Dave Parnaby, manager of my Middlesbrough side, asks what size shoes I wear, it sounds as if I'm being cut before a ball's even been kicked. Thankfully someone else brought a spare pair, meaning we didn't need to rummage through the Spennymoor lost and found box.

Dave stands to make a speech. He tells us to treat it like any other game. Don't be afraid to let the ball go up in the air. Don't be frightened to launch it long. Don't be scared to swing in crosses. After all, today is about seeing how those sorts of situations are handled when heads cannot be used. 'No problem, gaffer,' is the collective response. There are chaps here who know what's it like to be knocked out, cut open a head, break a nose. They're as intrigued as anyone to see how this goes.

It's 2.55pm now. T-minus five minutes, and naturally I'm nervous. Michael Barron, a hero of mine who I grew up watching as a Hartlepool United season ticket holder, asks if I've ever played with professionals before. I haven't, and his widening eyes don't fill me with confidence. We walk out of the tunnel and, bizarrely, because of injuries, the Middlesbrough bench has a population of one: me, the not-so-super sub. The Spennymoor bench consists of five, by comparison.

The winner will take home the Bill Gates Celebration Cup. I didn't know Bill when he was Bill, and what I mean by that is I've only met the man he is now. Over the course of a morning spent at his charming home in Castle Eden, County Durham, a few weeks prior to this match, Bill barely said a word. Whereas once he might have led the conversation, now he likes to listen, with his brain no longer able to keep up. Formerly a centre-back, Bill made more than 350 appearances as a professional but retired from playing at the age of 30 after being plagued by migraines. Now in his 70s, he's living with probable Chronic Traumatic Encephalopathy – 'probable' because CTE can only be confirmed by post-mortem examination. His wife, Dr Judith Gates, is the co-founder of Head for Change. 'Bill used to say when he was in his 30s, 40s and 50s that he would develop dementia one day,' she says, looking over at her husband as the light threatens to sneak through the clouds and into their conservatory. 'It was based on him estimating that he headed 100 balls a day in training. Bill was never knocked unconscious but he did take the occasional blow. I have a picture of him being given smelling salts during a game. Bill saw the generation before him develop dementia. He saw it coming for him, too, and he was right. He's lost his essence. When diagnosed, we made two promises together, Bill and I. One was that we'd optimise his life. The other was that as part of his legacy, we'd try to protect other players going forward.'

Bill's final season as a footballer was in 1973/74. He had to think carefully about the decision to retire prematurely because that was the campaign in which Jack Charlton's Middlesbrough were promoted to the First Division. There was an offer of another contract. He could have stayed and been a top-flight footballer but the migraines were too much. 'The concern is in 30 years' time, somebody will be sitting in a chair like I am now and saying the same things about football being dangerous,' Dr Gates adds. Head for Change wanted to make clear that the aim of this test run in Spennymoor was not to insist that heading should be outlawed. It was to kick-start a discussion which was long overdue and raise awareness of the risks. 'The brain doesn't know what's insulted it,' she says. 'It just knows it's been insulted.'

At 2.57pm, we're gathered around the centre circle. 'Bill Gates, ladies and gentlemen,' says Andy Sixsmith, the man with the mic. Bill shuffles to the centre, flanked by his son, Nick. There's a minute's applause – a mark of respect for those claimed by dementia and cancer, with this match raising money for both afflictions. As we applaud, Bill spies the match ball by his feet. He gives it a kick, for old times' sake, and it rolls a few inches. He smiles, as if transported back in time.

Applause over, it's 3pm, and time to kick off this footballing first. There have been a great number of variations of the game. The Chinese pastime of 'Tsu Chu' is credited by some to be the earliest form of football. Played more than 2,000 years ago, it involved teams trying to boot the ball into a silken net stretched between a pair of bamboo poles. Emperors took it seriously – to the extent that one minister who dared to suggest it was an unseemly exercise in AD 881 was sentenced to death. 'On the emperor's birthday two teams played football before the royal pavilion,' state records. 'The winners were rewarded with fruit, flowers and wine, with silver cups and brocaded hats. The captain of the losing side was flogged and made to suffer much indignity.' Thankfully there would be no such repercussions from this match, no matter how poorly I play.

That early header by Mark Tinkler would be the only infringement of the entire game. 'When you've played the game and when the ball's there to be headed, you go up to win it,' he later said in his defence. 'It's instinctive.' For the first half, we could use our heads inside of the penalty area and that was how the opening goal was scored – a fine finish at the back post by James Marwood, son of Brian, the former Arsenal and Hull City winger. Maybe that was football's dark sense of humour showing itself, a header commencing this game of no heading. Another comical moment cropped up when the ball was accidentally booted into the stands and a ten-year-old boy responded by heading it back into play. His father, slightly embarrassed, would explain the irony when he's old enough to understand.

The tie started with Middlesbrough taking a 2-0 lead and Spennymoor making it 2-2, Gavin Cogdon equalising from the penalty spot after a push in Carl Beasley's back. A controversial call, and not only because I'm the one who was apparently too rough in competing for the cross with Carl. In the Middlesbrough changing room, the chatter at half-time is about the soft decision. Meanwhile, out on the field, Dr Gates is addressing the crowd. 'My husband, Bill, will enjoy the game today,' she says, 'but he won't remember it tomorrow.' Before the start of the second half, we're reminded that there is no heading allowed whatsoever. That rule isn't broken once as Spennymoor take a 4-2 lead before Middlesbrough make it 5-4. The final score is 5-5 and the subsequent penalty shoot-out won by Spennymoor, with Craig Hignett's cheeky attempt at a Panenka punished. 'It was good fun, but the main point of the day was to raise awareness about dementia in football,' says Dave Parnaby. That it did, and it wasn't a bore draw. It was an entertaining, exciting, we lead, you lead tie. Ten goals, only one of them a header.

Did it still feel like football? Absolutely. When on the field, you didn't overthink the fact that you weren't allowed to use your head. You adjusted. You chested the ball instead of heading it. You trusted your passing ability. You tried to play your way into the opposition box. When heading wasn't allowed whatsoever, you crossed low and into the space in front of the forwards, with one such ball resulting in a tidy side-footed finish from Tommy Andrew. 'Good game, that,' was the consensus of the Middlesbrough changing room afterwards, coupled with surprise at how comfortable it felt. My team-mate Steve Howey, capped four times by England, admits he tries not to think about football's dementia problem now that he's in his 50s. It does concern him, though, particularly when words escape him mid-conversation.

It was fun to play in, but what did it look like from the stands? For that I defer to outside opinions. 'In the first half, in particular, you barely noticed the difference,' wrote Luke Edwards in the *Daily Telegraph*. 'In the second half, the change to the rules was far more apparent and, in truth, the spectacle suffered. With no heading allowed, there was too much short passing and it made defending easier without the threat of high crosses from the flanks. It was too much like five-a-side football.' Rod Liddle of *The Times* said something similar. 'Aside from the obvious observation – that it begins to resemble five-a-side football – the lack of headers tilts the game in favour of the defenders,' he wrote. 'Corners become pretty much pointless. So, too, those free kicks in which the player is urged to "shove it in the mixer". There is no mixer any more. But in time, surely, the players and the laws will adapt – because a ban on heading cannot be far away now.'

Mixed reviews, then, with a preference for the half when heading was still allowed in the two 18-yard boxes. Whether you're a fan of these tweaks or not, this experiment was evidence of why football's authorities can have few excuses for sitting idly by and not setting up one of their own. Theirs would need to be much more comprehensive than a one-off game played in the sun in Spennymoor, of course. Ideally it would last as long as a season and be studied, with players and fans providing feedback. Governing bodies such as the Football Association could see whether any divisions lower down the pyramid would want to participate in potentially the most significant trial in football history. Given the right incentive there would be volunteers, whether to test the game without any heading at all or with headers only permitted in the penalty areas.

Arsenal 'Invincible' Martin Keown tells me he would leave the pitch disappointed if he knew another player had won more headers than him. That was his own little contest. Defenders like Martin spent their careers clearing the danger by any means. So what happens when you limit those means? Well, let's see. Let's see if we miss those commanding clearances. Let's see if we don't mind the game without those glancing headers. Let's see if some clever coach finds a way to exploit the situation, such as by telling his team to float balls in behind for his streak-of-lightning striker. Let's see if this creates chaos from long balls and let's see if we like that. Until trialled properly, we will never know for sure.

Dr Judith Gates is disappointed but glad. Disappointed this hasn't happened yet. Glad they could get the conversation started with this Spennymoor test run. She mentions her great-grandson, Liam. He's three years old and recently learned a new word – 'delicate'. He's got a younger brother, Luca, who he daren't pick up. She asked him why, and Liam pointed to his sibling's head. 'He said "delicate",' says Dr Gates. 'That sums it up nicely, don't you think?'

8

# The Old Leather Ball Myth

*That 21st-century ball sitting in the centre circle*
*this Saturday doesn't do damage? Balls to that*

IT'S BECAUSE of that old leather ball, right? It *looked* heavy,
therefore it was. The modern-day ball *looks* light, therefore it is.
Not exactly. Let me explain.

On 31 March 1866, two teams made up of players from
London and Sheffield met at Battersea Park. The fixture was
described as the first of any importance under the auspices of the
Football Association and a size five ball was used, manufactured
by Lillywhites Ltd. Lining up for the victorious Londoners that
day was a 23-year-old called Charles Alcock who, soon enough,
would be one of English football's most influential figures. He
became FA secretary and on 20 July 1871, at a meeting held
in the offices of *The Sportsman* newspaper, this now suited-up
28-year-old had a suggestion. He had been educated at the
prestigious Harrow School and recalled playing in an inter-
house competition. The FA could and should create something
similar, he said. A contest in which all of their member clubs
compete for one trophy. The committee liked the idea and with
that, a new competition was born. The minutes of the meeting
state as much, 'That it is desirable that a Challenge Cup should
be established in connection with the Association for which all

clubs belonging to the Association should be invited to compete.' Today that competition is known as the FA Cup. When writing up the rules they needed a regulation ball, so they went with 'Lillywhites No 5', the same one used in that fixture between London and Sheffield.

Before this, there had been no specifications about the size of the ball. Only its shape, as stated in the lyrics to the old 'Brighton College Football Song', 'And Eton may play with a pill if they please, and Harrow may stick to their Cheshire cheese, and Rugby their outgrown egg, but here is the perfect game of the perfect sphere.' Soon football would have an idea of how big this 'sphere' should be, and how much it must weigh.

In 1889, the Laws of the Game specified its features in full for the first time – it should be between 27 and 28in in circumference, and from 12 to 15oz in weight. Contrary to popular belief, the balls used in today's Premier League matches aren't lighter than those of the 19th and 20th centuries. They can be heavier. The Laws for 2021, for example, listed the ball's latest specifics – between 27 and 28in, and from 14 to 16oz. So those artefacts sitting in the cabinets of the National Football Museum in Manchester, made of leather and with laces on the outside, were not automatically heavier than those of today. Not the one used between England and Wales in Wrexham on 11 March 1912. Nor the one used in the inaugural World Cup Final between Uruguay and Argentina on 30 July 1930. At 3pm this Saturday, that 21st-century ball you see sitting in the centre circle can weigh four ounces more than those used back in the day.

It was in 1937 when the ball's weight bracket was upped to 14 to 16oz and it has stayed that way since. One problem, though: in games played on wet and muddy afternoons, a ball made of authentic leather could and would become heavier. And let's face it, England can be a pretty soggy place. That's why for more than a century, the Laws have included a caveat – 'at the commencement of the game' or 'at the start of the match' – when specifying the ball's weight. It may have started at 14oz, or 16. But that would change once the heavens opened. In an experiment conducted on such an evening, it was found that the leather ball could gain 3oz in weight over the course of a match. Former Manchester United goalkeeper Gary Bailey was one of many encouraged to lump it long at every opportunity, as befitting the era. He says it was 'like kicking a piece of concrete'. Hoofing it wasn't easy when wet. Heading it wasn't fun, either.

On 8 March 1947, Wolverhampton Wanderers drew 1-1 at Middlesbrough in a First Division match played in difficult conditions. The ball became a lump and Stan Cullis, the legendary centre-back for Wolves, felt the repercussions. In his 1960 autobiography, *All For The Wolves*, you will find a photograph of Stan lying in a hospital bed at Sheffield Royal Infirmary, a nurse lifting a glass of water to his mouth. 'I was taken off the train from Middlesbrough with concussion after heading a heavy ball frequently,' he writes. 'It was this incident which caused me to decide to retire at the age of 31.' The Sheffield doctor was not the first to warn Stan that he should stop playing. The repercussions of heading had been weighing heavy on his mind, for lack of a better term, and so he decided it was finally time to heed the advice.

Stan went on to enjoy a fine career as a coach following his premature retirement as a player, winning three English championships with Wolves. Yet his final years were spent in a nursing home. Diagnosed with dementia, he could no longer attend fixtures at his beloved Molineux, respond to fan mail or recall his finest footballing moments with any real clarity. That includes the memory of how, at the tender age of 22, he became England's youngest-ever captain in an international friendly against Romania on 24 May 1939. 'When my dad went into a care home, he was always very grateful and gentle,' his son, Andrew, tells me, 'which I know is not the case for everyone with dementia.'

One peculiarity of the disease is how, through the fog, some of that person's past can still shine through. For many, music is the trigger. For my grandad, Robert Rowland, it was 'Blueberry Hill' by Fats Domino. He might not remember the names of relatives, or what he had for breakfast, but he could defy his dementia by singing that favourite song of his, from start to finish. For Stan, it was the language he'd learned at night school more than half a century earlier. 'In his teens, he had learnt Esperanto,' continues Andrew. 'In the care home, he could recite some Esperanto from all those years ago with great fluency.' On 28 February 2001, aged 84, Stan died. His family had long feared his memory loss and minor strokes were consequences of days spent heading tough leather. Stan's daughter, Susan, wrote to football's authorities about this concern but she received no response.

Clubs were completely aware that the ball would increase in weight when wet, too, and some would sneakily try to use this to their advantage allegedly. The final section of Bryony Hill's book about her husband, *My Gentleman Jim*, is titled 'The Hijacking of a Brain'. There she claims one of Jimmy's old clubs would soak the ball in a bucket of water overnight before a home game, causing it to increase in weight considerably. The idea was the away team would be expecting a 'normal' ball so this gave the hosts an edge of sorts. 'Can it therefore be purely coincidental,' she asks, 'that so many ex-professional footballers have developed dementia? Was it caused by the constant heading of these heavy balls?'

This was an issue when the Laws of the Game stated that the 'outer casing of the ball must be of leather'. But as technology advanced, so too did this ruling. Synthetic materials were given the go-ahead in the 1960s and with that, balls could be waterproofed. They could stay a constant weight, no matter the weather. This transition was the subject of an article in *The Guardian* on 28 November 1969, headlined 'From Sodden Leather to Polka Dots'. It explained how there was now a generation of footballers who would never play with the 'old-fashioned' leather ball which, according to the author, could leave players 'physically nauseated by the constant impact'.

Football wasn't immediate in switching to a non-absorbent synthetic shell, mind. In 1965, manufacturers were invited to make submissions for the official match ball of the 1966 World Cup. It led to 114 entrants which were then whittled down to eight in a blind test conducted in London. FIFA had the final say as tournament organisers, selecting the Slazenger Challenge 4-Star. Crafted by 32-year-old Malcolm Wainwright of Dewsbury, Yorkshire, it consisted of 25 hand-stitched leather panels and was bright orange in colour.

It was this ball which would cross the line four times for England in the final – three if you ask any Germans who still don't believe *that* strike by Sir Geoff Hurst should have counted. Sir Geoff didn't get to keep the ball with which he bagged a hat-trick. It transpired that Helmut Haller, who opened the scoring for West Germany, took it home with him after his country's 4-2 defeat. He had sneaked it back in his suitcase and given it as a gift to his son, Jürgen, on his fifth birthday. It took 30 years and a campaign by the *Daily Mirror* for the ball to be returned to its rightful owner. Helmut, to his credit, turned down the offer of a fat cheque and instead gave it back to Sir Geoff in exchange for a donation to a children's cancer charity.

During the ball's three decades in Germany, the game transitioned away from the use of leather. The 1986 World Cup in Mexico saw the first fully synthetic ball used. Adidas Azteca, it was named, with Diego Maradona getting a feel for it that day at the Estadio Azteca in Mexico City when he leapt with his left arm against England.

The 'old leather ball' myth is one which has long irritated Professor Willie Stewart, the world leader on brain disease in football. He considers it a way of kicking this problem 30, 40, potentially 50 years into the future. 'To say, "It's a disease of a bygone age. We're only seeing it in people who played 40 years ago." Well that's because of the nature of the disease,' says Prof Stewart. 'Of course we don't see it in the 23-year-olds currently playing. They're not old enough yet. Then what happens is people say, "Well if it's a disease of a former era, is there something we can blame it on? That might give us the comfort in believing it's gone away." And so, it's the old leather balls.' Prof Stewart's FIELD study focused on 7,676 former footballers born between 1 January 1900 and 1 January 1977, comparing them to 23,028 matched members of the general public. In separating those born between 1910 and 1929, 1930 and 1949, and 1950 and 1969, they recorded no radical changes. 'Risk of neurodegenerative disease,' the study stated, 'remained similar across players born in an era when solely leather balls would be used to players born in an era when there was a transition from leather to synthetic balls.'

It was enough to spark suggestions that balls sold in shops today should come with a cigarette-style health warning on the packaging, similar to what you'd see on a pack of Marlboro Gold. 'Warning: repeated heading of this ball can lead to increased risk of brain damage,' for example. Speak to scientists and campaigners and they will tell you they are afraid. The fear is there are ticking time bombs out there and that this will continue to grip future generations of footballers. Only then will it sink in that it wasn't all down to that 'leather lump'. Kevin Moore was the first known Premier League player to die after developing Pick's disease, also known as frontotemporal dementia. He was 55. Those close to the former defender cannot help fearing it was death by football, and most of Kevin's career was spent playing with a ball that was solely synthetic.

Frank McLintock, the captain of Arsenal's 1971 Double-winning side, likens heading the old ball to being hit by former heavyweight champion Sonny Liston. It doesn't gain weight when wet. It isn't a magnet to mud. But the modern ball can pack a punch, too. Just ask Matt Bloomfield. He is the former Wycombe Wanderers captain whose career was ended by a ball to the back of the head sustained during a goalless draw with Exeter City on 10 August 2021. A quick free kick was taken but the attempt at launching it long wasn't successful. It smacked Matt from close range and he was concussed. He had a history of head injuries and this time, the symptoms didn't want to disappear. He took his youngest daughter, Rosie, on the teacups at Peppa Pig World a month later and couldn't shake the dizziness. Doctors advised Matt to retire and he listened, meaning that trip to Exeter was his 558th and final appearance in a Wycombe shirt.

Prior to the millennium, the fastest shot recorded in a Premier League fixture was by Manchester United's David Beckham, clocked at 97.9mph against Chelsea on 22 February 1997. The book *Football Confidential* was an investigative look at the beautiful game. Its authors told the stories the authorities didn't want telling. One chapter revealed the ruthlessness of agents who were signing up starlets then binning them when they didn't make it big. Another detailed the dreadful pitches that were injuring hundreds of footballers. The book also looked at 'the link between football and Alzheimer's'. In that chapter, they took the Gadd Severity Index – the tool used by automotive manufacturers to measure the potential severity of head injury in a car crash – and applied it to football. Readers were told an index reading of 1,000 would result in severe concussion and, had a head stopped it, David Beckham's shot would have registered 300.

On 6 April 2008, a shot by Cristiano Ronaldo missed its target and instead flew into the stands of the Riverside Stadium. It made a beeline for Middlesbrough supporter Fred Harrison, who protected his face with his hands. He succeeded in stopping his glasses from breaking but only broke something else. The Manchester United man's attempt was struck so fiercely that it fractured this 68-year-old grandfather's right wrist. The ball swerved in the air and then Fred felt its power. It may float like a butterfly, but it stings like a bee, to borrow the iconic quote from Muhammad Ali.

Published in the *Scandinavian Journal of Medicine & Science in Sports* on 2 September 2020 was a study of the ball and the biomechanics of heading. It found 'force experienced by the head during heading is influenced more by speed than the mechanical properties of the football'. Using the MADYMO ellipsoid human body model – a computerised crash test dummy, in other words – researchers looked at speed versus mass versus stiffness. 'We wanted to understand what would be the best way to reduce the forces involved in football heading,' says Gregory Tierney, one of those behind the study. While keeping the other variables the same, they tested 4.5mph, then 8.9mph, then 13.4mph, and so on, all the way up to 53.7mph, which is believed to be the greatest speed at which a defender will head a goal kick back in the opposite direction. They then applied the same method in terms of mass. Then of stiffness. From that they came to a conclusion. 'What this gave us was that initial indication that the speed of the ball is the main contributor to the forces felt by the head,' adds Gregory, who says they are aiming to find out more. 'We only looked at modern balls, which are mainly elastic in their nature, whereas the older balls likely have different material properties. We would like to answer that question. The sad reality of research is the answer at the end is usually that more is needed. But we're hoping to get started soon.'

The ball's bite has been demonstrated by other studies, too. One in 2015 which found the forces generated from heading a goal kick were similar to those from a tackle in American football. Another in 2016 which said a typical heading practice session can lead to immediate impairment in brain function. Likewise it has been highlighted that if you double the mass of the ball, you double the kinetic energy. If you double the speed, you quadruple it.

Edmund Waller, the English poet, was once inspired into writing about how football enthusiasts would make use of the beasts they butchered at Christmas. 'And now in winter when men kill the fat swine, they get the bladder and blow it great,' he wrote, adding, 'While it is thrown and caste up in the ayre, each one contendeth and hath a great delite.'

The oldest ball in existence was made of a pig's bladder, with laces protruding. It is currently housed in a glass cabinet at the Stirling Smith Art Gallery and Museum. Discovered in the ceiling panelling of the Queen's Chamber in Stirling Castle, Scotland, its origin remains a mystery. Some believed it was bought by King James IV, with accounts showing he purchased a bag of four 'fut ballis' for two shillings in 1497. Others claim it belonged to Mary, Queen of Scots, who was a fan of football, so say records. The likeliest reason for how it was originally lost is that during King James V's reconstruction of the castle from 1537, it was booted so high that it became lodged in the rafters. And there it remained as a result of that overzealous kick until its discovery in 1969. Looking at it, you wouldn't fancy your chances of curling it around a four-man wall. Football has come a long way since a pig's bladder was used for a game between pals at the park.

The balls of today are designed to be as sensitive to the player's touch as possible and their descriptions are packed with scientific jargon about RaDaR visual technology, Aerowtrack grooves, how its 3D printed ink overlay fine-tunes its flight, how its 12-panel fuse-welded synthetic leather casing gives its users maximum control. It is terminology which wouldn't look unusual in a NASA manual. They fly through the air – albeit not off the shelves at a cost of £124.95 for the same one used in Premier League fixtures – and they're only getting faster.

The Nike Geo Merlin, with which Sir Alex Ferguson's Manchester United were crowned champions in 2000/01, was billed as the 'roundest, fastest, most accurate ball ever'. The Nike Total 90 Aerow I, with which Jose Mourinho's Chelsea won their first title in 2004/05, had a 'greater speed' after more than 100 hours of laboratory tests. In 2014/15 we had the Nike Ordem 2, described as being perfect for anything from 'supple first touches to mind-bending, powerful shots'. In 2020/21 we had the Nike Flight, billed as 'fused for power' after being 'honed over eight years and 1,700 hours of testing'. It is why that study which suggested speed is the greatest factor in the force absorbed by the head should be a concern.

An afternoon in the company of Paul Gascoigne at his home in Poole led to talk of how he fell in love with football, long before he became an England icon. It all started with a gift. Not the God-given one which helped him score against Scotland at Euro '96, but a gift given to him by his dad, John. 'I got my first-ever ball off him when I was seven,' said the man who could do magical things with it. 'I dribbled with it to school, dribbled it home, headed it, slept with it.' Momentarily lost in that era, Paul's eyes welled up. 'All the time. It was football, morning and night.' Smiling, he then turned his attention to his mum, Carol. 'My mam used to say, "Right, son, get to bed." I'd go to bed, but then I'd climb down the drainpipe so I could play football in the street.' And she didn't have a clue? 'Did she f***, until the pipe broke.' With you on it? 'Aye! Boomf. My mam wasn't happy. She was like John Wayne with a slipper – she never missed!'

That ball was practically a friend to a young Paul. Many footballers hold similarly romantic stories about their first. You might even remember yours. I know I do, having lost mine to the rooftop of an amusement arcade in Seaton Carew, Hartlepool. It is memories like Paul's which can make it difficult to believe that this little companion of ours could be a health hazard.

Count the headers in the 1966 World Cup Final and you'll see that there were a total of 103 between England and West Germany. There were 106 between the English and Germans when they met at Euro 2020 by comparison. Heading is by no means obsolete. Sometimes a striker might head the ball repeatedly during a match, sometimes not at all. Sir Geoff Hurst says he would practise on a Monday, Tuesday, Wednesday, Thursday and Friday, all with the aim of making it count on the Saturday. It worked that day at Wembley when he equalised using his head in the 18th minute. England became world champions with a leather ball. But those synthetic ones of today are as heavy and, thanks to technological advances, they're faster, too. They think it's all over. Really, this might be as big of a problem now as it was back then.

9

# 'The Invisible Patients'

*How female footballers are potentially more at risk
than men and yet have been overlooked*

WORLDWIDE, WOMEN with dementia outnumber men two
to one and yet this cohort have been grossly under-represented
when it comes to investigating brain damage in sport. Research
is rarely female focused, though that which has been conducted
has produced concerning results. One study called 'Association
of Sex with Adolescent Soccer Concussion Incidence and
Characteristics', for example, looked at 43,741 male footballers
against 39,637 female between 2016 and 2019 in America. It
found girls were almost twice as likely to be concussed as boys –
1.88 times, to be precise – while they also took longer to recover.
Since 2015, every high school in the state of Michigan has entered
data into the 'Head Injury Reporting System'. If a student is
suspected of concussion, it's recorded in this database. That was
the source of this study's statistics, and the cause of each injury was
likewise logged. It could be noted as 'person-to-person contact',
such as a clash of heads, or 'person-to-object contact', like heading
the ball. Whereas the most common mechanism of concussion
among men was the former, for women it was the latter.

These findings corresponded with the experience of Sue
Lopez. Hers isn't a name as recognised as Wayne Rooney's or Gary
Lineker's, but this former forward is one of the most iconic figures

in English football history. On 27 January 2020, in an interview with the BBC, Sue became the first female player to publicly link her condition to her career. When picturing dementia in football, you might think of the goalscorer who cannot remember a single one of his goals. The captain who forever knew what to say in his team talks but now words fail him. The winger who delighted in dazzling supporters but now his days are spent in a care home, awaiting the end. All accurate, though the key word in each of those examples is 'his'. Sue wanted the world to know this wasn't just happening to men. It was happening to women, too. 'I think the dementia – my dementia – has been caused by the heading of the ball,' said this icon in her 70s.

In her prime, Sue represented Southampton and Roma and won 22 caps for England. She later coached for the Hampshire Football Association and was awarded the MBE in 2000 for services to women's football. Flanked by her best friend and former team-mate Lesley Lloyd, Sue is asked who gave her that MBE. 'I don't remember.' Prince Charles, perhaps? 'It was obviously before the dementia.' It's known that the number in men's football is three-and-a-half times – that's how much more likely professional players are to die with neurodegenerative disease than the common man. There's no number for women in football to go by. Not yet.

Sue has deteriorated since that BBC interview. She doesn't talk much today but she's fortunate to have a friend in Lesley, who will speak up for her. Women's football wasn't always so welcomed by the powers that be. There was a time when it was given the red card, so to speak. 'Complaints having been made as to football being played by women,' read a statement from the Football Association on 5 December 1921, 'the Council feel impelled to express their strong opinion that the game of football is quite unsuitable for females and ought not to be encouraged.' From this, Football League grounds were prohibited from hosting women's fixtures. It wasn't until 1971 that this ban was lifted and that same year, Sue and Lesley won the inaugural women's FA Cup Final for Southampton, beating Stewarton Thistle 4-1 on a bobbly pitch at the Crystal Palace National Sports Centre. Forward Sue and captain Lesley together lifted the Mitre Challenge Trophy, as it was called for sponsorship purposes at the time. They were the first women to do so.

It may be a one-sided conversation between these two pioneers these days owing to Sue's dementia, but Lesley visits her friend's care home near the historic Hampshire village of Botley whenever she can. 'I saw Marieanne Spacey – the manager of Southampton – the other day and I told her that she sends her love and regards,' Lesley tells me. 'But Sue was blank. Absolutely blank. Sometimes I don't know if she even knows who I am any more. It's awful to watch. But I've got photos on my mobile phone. We used to walk llamas! Show her one of those and her face will light up. She's never lost her love of animals. I talk to her about football, about the past, what we did, what we achieved, but I don't get a lot back.' Lesley pauses. 'You know what dementia is like.'

Sue was ahead of her time. As a player, she didn't think heading was good for her health, though it was somewhat unavoidable. 'To get into the England team, she was told she had to head the ball,' adds Lesley. 'It sounds silly but she had to do it, so she'd spend hours having a ball thrown or kicked at her. She once went to a doctor with concussion after being knocked flat. He said, "Oh, you should be doing something far more suitable for a lady!" She just laughed. It wasn't taken seriously back then. It just wasn't.' As a coach, Sue wouldn't impose this sort of practice on her players, not wishing to expose them to the same trauma she endured. 'She was very thorough. Whoever she was coaching, she'd set out a plan for the session the night before, and it didn't involve heading, I can tell you that. If they didn't need to do it, why do it? That's what she thought. We played together in the early '70s. In all the time I've known her, she's always said, "I don't want them – children – heading the ball." She was so adamant. She had a football brain and she knew, from her own experiences, that heading affects you, especially if you play for years and years. I played from 1968 to 1973. I married my husband, Graham, had two kids, Joanna and Alison, and that was the end of me playing football. But Sue played on. She's got all the awards – an honorary doctorate from the University of Southampton, the MBE, goodness knows what else – but her concern, even at 74 years old, was for other people heading the ball.'

That's why Sue decided to speak up in that BBC interview, while she still could. Four weeks later, the FA announced it was banning under-12s from practising heading in training. A beneficial ban this time, unlike that one issued in 1921. 'It was a big step for Sue to say what she said,' says Lesley. 'I like to tell her she changed the world.' Certainly there are worse legacies to leave behind.

Michelle Akers, the United States great with 105 goals in 153 games and two-time winner of the Women's World Cup, is worried about her future, too. Now in her 50s, she has suffered from migraines and memory lapses. She isn't sure what's down to damage from football and what is merely a consequence of getting older. She doesn't know if she will be in the same situation as Sue in 20 years' time or free from dementia. Whatever happens, when she's gone, Michelle's brain will go to Boston University's CTE Centre and so will her former US team-mate Brandi Chastain's. 'It is really about how I can help impact soccer beyond scoring a goal in 1999 in the World Cup Final,' Brandi said after announcing her decision to donate. 'Can I do something more to leave soccer in a better place than it was when I began this wonderful journey with this game?'

Why women are so much more at risk of concussion remains the subject of research. Scientists have speculated it is potentially due to physical and physiological differences between the sexes. What happens when a human being is concussed is an incredibly complex process but one the 2014 documentary *Head Games: The Global Concussion Crisis* tried to explain using Play-Doh. Your brain is connected by nerve fibres called axons. They're about one micrometre in diameter – that's 100 times thinner than a human hair – and yet it is this wiring which connects that vast network of neurons we're all carrying upstairs. When stretched slowly, that lump of Play-Doh will move but stay intact. Stretch it at speed, however, and it will break. It is this violent action which can harm or kill the axons, sometimes causing them to disconnect from the cells to which they're supposed to stay attached. With that, you're concussed.

Scientists from Philadelphia previously found females have more fragile and breakable nerve fibres compared to males – potentially explaining why they're at a greater risk of concussion and can have extended recovery periods. Other researchers have speculated it's due to our differing hormones, or to do with the strength of neck muscles. Theories such as these are still being examined. What is known is when our nerves die as a result of repetitive concussive or subconcussive blows, there's neurodegeneration in later life. The SCORES study – short for Screening Cognitive Outcomes after Repetitive head impact Exposure in Sport and led by Dr Michael Grey – is investigating this long-term effect. It involves former athletes, male and female and including footballers, over the age of 40 being assessed every three months for the next ten years of their lives via online tests. The idea is Dr Grey and his colleagues at the University of East Anglia can use this data to detect any subtle changes in brain function as these men and women age.

Lingering like a bad smell in football is a macho mentality, telling you it's weak to want to leave that field. This mindset was found to be a major reason why 78.7 per cent of sportsmen said they had played through concussion in a 2016 investigation conducted in the United States. 'You don't tap out in Texas high school or college football unless you have to,' said one of the 843 athletes involved in the study. 'It was considered unmanly,' answered another. No guts, no glory, and all that. This is not an exclusive mentality among men, however. That same survey found 69.1 per cent of sportswomen failed to report their concussion, too, instead choosing to play on.

It would be wrong to think of women's football as, for lack of a better term, 'girly'. It's blood and thunder. It's broken bones and battle scars. It's elite-level competitiveness and Faye White, the former Arsenal Ladies defender and England's longest-serving captain, has felt it. The nose break at the 2007 World Cup. The cheekbone fracture at Euro 2009 – the final of which she played wearing a Phantom of the Opera-esque face mask as protection. The two anterior cruciate ligament injuries which kept her away from the Arsenal defence for longer than she would have liked. When injured, Faye would largely have to fend for herself, overseeing her own recovery. That's just the way it was, for her and everyone else. 'Should my knee feel this way?' 'Am I overdoing it?' 'Should I be training today?' All questions women have asked themselves throughout their footballing careers, including Faye.

Faye was fortunate in that she could occasionally consult Colin Lewin, the physiotherapist who treated the men's squad from 1995 until 2018. In the absence of full-time care for the women's side, Colin chipped in, his good relationship with manager Vic Akers assisting that crossover. 'Vic would say, "Look, we've got a tricky one here, would you mind giving us an opinion?"' Colin recalls. Thankfully the operation at the

Women's Super League club is much more professional today. Arsenal Ladies now have a full-time physio in place and Gary Lewin, Colin's cousin, was named their head of medicine and sports science ahead of the 2021/22 WSL season – in what was a new role created by the club. 'When you think women's footballers now have access to psychologists, nutritionists, physios, doctors, without having to go off-site, without having to lean on the men's team, it's great,' Colin says. 'I'm not saying they get the same facilities and I don't think they get the same therapist-to-player ratio – the budgets are different – but it's come on enormously over the last ten years and so it should.'

Colin is right to mention the contrasting budgets. That's reflected in the prize money they receive, like how the winners of the men's 2021/22 FA Cup earned £1.8m while the victorious women made only £25,000, the equivalent of 1.4 per cent. Arsenal's hirings can only be good for a game that's getting bigger and better. Sadly not all clubs can afford to hire such medical support, however. Some footballers are still in the same situation as Faye all those years ago, tending to themselves by listening to their bodies and, in cases of concussion, their brains.

There have never been more women in football than there are today. It isn't the 'boys only' club it was previously portrayed to be. Far from it. Other fields have acknowledged their need to adapt. In the world of the Air Force, fighter jets were historically designed with male pilots in mind. The arm length required to reach the cockpit controls. The sitting height needed to see through the windshield. The minimum weight for the ejection seat to work. Everything was based on a 1967 survey of males. Because of this bias, female officers found themselves excluded. They didn't pass the physical standards and so couldn't fly that F-15 Eagle. This inequality is now being acknowledged and addressed, slowly but surely.

There is a debate over whether football should be considering changes, too. Changes which would be specific to women. Changes to the concussion protocols, which are currently based on male-dominated studies, or to how much heading is permitted in training. In a survey of 2,000 people conducted by Censuswide, on behalf of head injury charity The Drake Foundation, 84 per cent of the female footballers questioned said they would welcome limits. Some WSL clubs, including Manchester United Women, have already turned to virtual reality to reduce the trauma being taken on by their footballers. Developed by Rezzil, the VR headset allows players to practise heading without the impact. Users have praised the software for its realism. The *Daily Mail*'s women's football correspondent Kathryn Batte tested it out. 'It feels like you are really there in the box,' Kathryn says. 'So much so that when I turned and saw a ball flying towards me I ducked to avoid being hit in the face!'

It is partly because of sport's lack of sex-specific guidelines that PINK Concussions was founded by Katherine Snedaker. PINK is the world's first non-profit organisation focusing solely on female traumatic brain injury. It didn't start with a girl, however. It started with a boy. Specifically, Katherine's son, who was ten years old when concussion made him miss close to a year at Roton Middle School in Norwalk, Connecticut. 'I got a call to say that he'd been hit in the head by a soccer ball at recess,' she recalls of 27 October 2008. 'I had to pick him up and take him to the paediatrician.' The recovery process for this freak accident was anything but straightforward. Katherine heard the same advice, over and over again. 'Tell your son to rest until he's clear of symptoms,' it went. Waking up with a headache and going to bed with one, too? 'Rest.' Still happening a month later? 'Rest.' Two months later? 'Rest.' It was like Groundhog Day. The longer Katherine waited for her son's symptoms to clear, the sooner that guidance got old, as it would for any parent. His headaches might subside after a few months and he'd be allowed to return to school, then one blow to the head would bring him back to square one. 'Rest,' they would be told, again.

Frustrated, Katherine felt compelled to learn about what was happening to her son. She studied head injuries by reading books and scientific papers. She consulted experts. She attended conferences. She established support groups. In Norwalk – the coastal city an hour's drive from New York – Katherine became known as the 'concussion mom'. She was the parent to phone if your child was concussed and you wanted to know more. While working in two concussion clinics, Katherine noticed a trend – girls being taken to doctors days, sometimes weeks, later than boys and who were not healing as fast as their families, friends, teachers and coaches felt they should have been.

Sadly her work stopped when disaster struck twice in three months. First Katherine's home was partially destroyed by Hurricane Sandy, that Category 3 superstorm which devastated the north-eastern United States in October 2012. Then she was diagnosed with breast cancer in January 2013. Yet it was while undergoing chemotherapy and radiation therapy that she set up PINK. What started as an educational website in 2013 is now a fully fledged organisation focusing on female brain injury, helping any woman damaged by sport, domestic violence, military service or in an accident. For too long, Katherine says, women have been 'the invisible patients' of this 'invisible injury' and that's a problem.

Amid a flurry of reports on Chronic Traumatic Encephalopathy among male American footballers, Katherine wondered what research had been conducted on females. Here was a conveyor belt of men's brains being searched for tau protein – that toxic soup associated with CTE – but what about women? In searching for what studies had been conducted, she found two papers. One was from 1990 and called 'Dementia in a punch-drunk wife', detailing a 76-year-old woman who was abused at the hands of her husband. The beatings she endured left her with bruises, broken bones and, notably, 'cauliflower ears'. She grew demented and following her death, her brain was found to be like that of a boxer's. The other study was from 1991 and called 'Neuropathological observations in a case of autism presenting with self-injury behaviour'. This one told the story of a 24-year-old autistic girl. Hers was a troubled history which included repeatedly banging her head against walls. As a result, her brain looked like it was from the skull of a boxer.

And that's it. Two studies. It is worth noting that both of these women's brains were examined only by chance, Katherine explains. The 'punch-drunk wife' because this corpse with 'cauliflower ears' intrigued researchers who knew this was a trait of boxers. The 'autistic girl' because autism in women is rare compared to men. Katherine sought out the scientists behind these studies. While CTE was not named in either paper, Dr Patrick Hof, who led the examination of the woman with autism, told her he believes she had the trauma-induced disease.

Of the first 1,000 donors to the Brain Bank in Boston, only 28 were female compared to 972 male, and that's a staggering imbalance. Anyone who donates must overcome that 'ick' factor – the thought of their brain someday sitting on a slab in a laboratory, a knife slicing through it. Katherine's come to terms with that. As someone who's sustained concussions herself – at least 20, her first in a car crash at the age of 16 – she has committed to donating her brain after death. Hers will go to the Mount Sinai Brain Bank in New York. Michelle Akers' and Brandi Chastain's will go to Boston. Rose Reilly's will go to Glasgow, the woman who was crowned the world's best female footballer in 1984 having announced her desire to donate previously.

To finish, Katherine shows me a bar graph she created for a past presentation. It's called 'Sympathy measured in casseroles'. She made it for fun, but behind it is a serious message. When her divorce was finalised, a friend brought her a casserole. When Hurricane Sandy damaged her home, there were more well wishes and, of course, more casseroles. When diagnosed with breast cancer, she was swimming in food hampers, chocolates, flowers – more sympathy than she knew what to do with. Yet when she and her son were concussed, there was none of this. No casseroles. No checking in. 'We're taught with cancer to support each other,' Katherine concludes.

But not with concussion, and that's wrong. This is an injury which can leave you feeling like there's a clamp squeezing your skull. That cannot be underestimated. Nor can the fact that women are potentially more at risk than men. It could come courtesy of a clenched fist at home, as in the tragic tale of the 'punch-drunk wife'. Or in a car crash. Or on the battlefield. Or on the football field. However inflicted, those jolts to the head matter. They all add up. Just ask Sue Lopez.

# 10

# A Macho Mess

*Terry Butcher, bloodied shirts, and why footballers
never say die in this brawn–before–brain game*

MAYBE MUHAMMAD Ali standing over Sonny Liston.
Maybe Diego Maradona being confronted by six Belgians.
Maybe Michael Jordan flying through the air, about to dunk.
Maybe Usain Bolt somehow finding time in a 9.86s sprint in
the 100m semi-final at the 2016 Olympics to look to his left
and smirk. Plenty of pictures could claim to be the most iconic
captured in sporting history.

Another contender is the one of Terry Butcher, taken at
Stockholm's Rasunda Stadion on 6 September 1989 and which
earned its place in English football heritage. You know the
one. With his white shirt stained red and a bandage wrapped
around his temple, England's captain has just given blood for his
country. There was a high ball, a clash of heads with Sweden
striker Johnny Ekstrom, then five stitches at half-time. It wasn't
enough. More were needed but the second half was about to start
and there was no way he wasn't walking out of that tunnel with
his team-mates. England were on the verge of qualifying for
the 1990 World Cup so the team's doctor, John Crane, wrapped
Terry up as well as he could. Looking like Mr Bump, out he
went. With Terry's help, England earned a goalless draw, enough
to leave them well on their way to Italia '90. Joking around

afterwards, manager Sir Bobby Robson told reporters that his gladiatorial skipper actually required 22 stitches, so gaping was the wound. 'Terry's performance epitomised what he is all about,' said the boss. 'The boy is all heart and character.'

For years, wherever he managed, Terry would receive fan mail. Most of the envelopes would contain a copy of *that* picture with a request for him to sign and send back. A glance on eBay suggests a few of those fans were in the business of making money rather than collecting mementos. Looking back now, Terry feels it was 'foolish' of him to remain on the field and head ball after ball with almost reckless abandon. Staying on had nothing to do with bravery, he says, or being a lionheart. It was misguided machoism. He couldn't walk away, lest he be seen as weak or not a committed England captain.

He felt obliged to play on. 'I was losing a lot of blood,' Terry tells me, more than 30 years on from the night his head was split open in Stockholm. 'But I was captain of my country, it was a World Cup qualifier and your heart rules your head. I was raised in an era where if you shed some blood it was a badge of honour. You didn't think of the dangers. You thought of a broken leg. That was the worst injury that could happen to you. But when you think about it, a head collision – or brain trauma, which it is – is worse. If you broke your leg, you'd come off. But when you got a knock to your head, you'd carry on, unless you were *really* out of it.' Knowing what he knows now, like how vulnerable you are immediately after a head injury, Terry says it wasn't worth the risk of playing on. Not for the qualification point. Not for that snap of him in his bloodied shirt. Not for the 'Captain Blood' nickname which the Swedish media bestowed upon him. Not even for the six-month supply of washing powder he received from detergent brand Radion as a reward.

'I got back to the hotel after the game,' continues the former central defender, who was playing for Rangers under Graeme

Souness at the time. 'I had a glass of red wine. Several glasses, actually, because we'd drawn the game and it was a good point. This was on the Wednesday night. I flew back to Glasgow on Thursday, got home, didn't train, then on Friday went to training. Graeme said to me straightaway that morning, "Well done. You're playing tomorrow." That was it. Of course that was all I needed. I trained and I had an appointment to make a personal appearance [at a Nike store] at about 2pm. But I felt dizzy. I felt really, really, really out of it. I thought, "I have to go home and lie down." I thought I was going to pass out.' This was around 36 hours after the clash of heads with his Swedish opponent. 'That was when I felt the repercussions of that, on the Friday,' Terry continues. 'I went home, went to bed and didn't get up until the next morning.' He woke at 10am. Rangers were playing Scottish Premiership title rivals Aberdeen at Ibrox at 3pm. 'I played,' he says of that 1-0 win in front of 40,283 supporters. 'Speak to a neurosurgeon about that now and they'll shake their head. They'll say, "You idiot." But it was what it was.'

It's amazing what adrenalin can do. I myself have continued with a busted ankle, only for a visit to A&E at Charing Cross Hospital to later confirm it was broken. That was amateur football with little at stake. At the professional level, there's pride, pressure and a mortgage to pay. Some play through the pain because if they don't, they'll lose their win bonus, their place in the team and perhaps their chance of a new contract. Terry says the reason he refused to surrender was simple – he was brought up to believe being 'manly' was an unwritten rule of football, 'I remember watching Ipswich Town in 1978, beating West Bromwich Albion 3-1 in the FA Cup semi-final at Highbury. There was a clash between Brian Talbot and John Wile.' It saw blood spilled, shirts stained, stitches sewn and bandages wrapped around heads. 'In that era, it was expected of you to stay on,' says Terry, who was 19 years old when he witnessed this collision. 'If you came off, you were considered to be weak.'

Stockholm 1989 wasn't the only time Terry gave blood. Nor was it the first. He also did it on 23 January 1982 in the FA Cup fourth round against Luton Town. 'I broke my nose and played on,' he explains, 'despite blood pouring down the back of my throat. It was awful. I was sticky, choking on blood, but playing. My Ipswich team-mates were pleading with me but I stayed on because I was a kid and I wanted to impress. We went 3-0 up and only then did I decide it was time to come off.' You'd think what happened next would have acted as a warning when his England shirt was becoming a bloody rag against Sweden seven years later. 'I was in hospital for five weeks after that,' Terry adds. 'So I was pretty much used to blood.'

This determination to continue or die trying has been a theme since the game's start. Bert Trautmann was the Manchester City goalkeeper who broke his neck in the 1956 FA Cup Final after diving at the feet of Birmingham City's Peter Murphy. He didn't submit, though. He played on, making saves towards the end of the match and picking up a winners' medal at Wembley after a 3-1 win for City. The climb towards the Royal Box wasn't the best for Bert, with supporters' congratulatory slaps on the back sending painful shockwaves throughout his body. Footage shows him using his right hand to thank Her Majesty The Queen before returning it to his neck. 'Why is your head crooked?' Prince Philip asks. 'Stiff neck,' replies the goalkeeper, carrying his gloves under his armpit.

That was on the Saturday. It wasn't until the Tuesday that Bert, still in agony, went to Manchester Royal Infirmary. There an X-ray provided confirmation – a break so bad that doctors said he was lucky not to be paralysed, or worse. He had also, in all likelihood, suffered an almighty case of concussion. Certainly that's how it sounded when Bert recalled the aftermath, likening the collision to two trains colliding in a 2006 interview with *The Guardian* to mark the 50th anniversary of the final, 'It was such a strange sensation. I wasn't seeing any colour. Everything around me was grey and I couldn't see any of the players properly. I could only see silhouettes. It was like walking around in fog and trying to find my way. I can't remember what happened during the rest of the match.' Two months later he was holidaying near Munich, casting his fishing line into a creek with a brace around his neck and bandages around his head. He was the German who arrived in England as a prisoner of war but would become the first foreigner to be named Footballer of the Year. Yet Bert admitted later in life that the acclaim wasn't worth it, conceding he should have departed the field that day at Wembley on 5 May 1956, 'I carried on. People talk about bravery. But if I'd known my neck was broken I'd have been off like a shot.'

The term 'Wembley Hoodoo' was coined after a succession of FA Cup finals were spoiled by serious injuries. In 1955, Manchester City's Jimmy Meadows broke his leg – he didn't continue. In 1956, Bert broke his neck – he did. In 1957, Manchester United's Ray Wood broke his jaw – he did. In 1959, Nottingham Forest's Roy Dwight broke his leg – he didn't. In 1960, Blackburn Rovers' Dave Whelan broke his leg – he didn't. The lesson to take from all of this? If you could stand on two feet, you continued.

It didn't help that substitutes were only introduced into English football from 1965. Prior to this, an injured player departing the pitch would leave his team down to ten men. More often than not, therefore, they would play on – even if they endured a broken neck or jaw, it seems. It was a brawn-before-brain game, and there have been enough examples of footballers continuing after head injuries to suggest that seeing stars isn't a sufficient excuse for succumbing. Sometimes smelling salts would encourage players to come to their senses. Sometimes a simple pat-down would suffice. 'Man with the magic sponge' read one headline after the death of former England coach Harold Shepherdson, who even released a book called *The Magic Sponge*. 'Some of the games were laughable,' Sir Geoff Hurst says of his era. 'If I was knocked over, I'd want to get up again and show I wasn't hurt.' Mercifully, on 21 August 1965, after the Football Association reluctantly approved substitutes, Charlton Athletic's Keith Peacock became the first one used in a Football League game. But the desire to defy your injury was already ingrained in football. The use of a 12th man wasn't about to change that culture. It still exists today.

Some contests were savage, too, such as Chelsea against Leeds United in the replay of the 1970 FA Cup Final. This was a match of absolute aggression, described as 'the most brutal game in English football history' by the BBC. In 1997, former Premier League referee David Elleray reviewed the footage and said he would have shown six red cards. In 2020, Michael Oliver said he would have issued 11. Eric Jennings showed a solitary yellow card on the day. 'At times, it appeared that Mr Jennings would give a free kick only on production of a death certificate,' wrote Hugh McIlvanney, the doyen of sportswriting. Well, what else would you expect with players such as Ron 'Chopper' Harris and Norman 'Bites Yer Legs' Hunter in the line-ups? Peter Bonetti was clobbered by Mick Jones. Peter Osgood kneed by Jack Charlton. Billy Bremner kung-fu kicked by Eddie McCreadie. Years later, Eddie Gray stood up to make a speech at a dinner. Ron Harris was in the audience. 'I'd like to make a special presentation to "Chopper",' he said, holding up a screw-in stud from the bottom of a boot. 'I took it out of my kneecap all those years ago.' There was one substitution in this 1970 final – a tactical change by Chelsea manager Dave Sexton in extra time as he replaced a striker with a defender to protect their 2-1 lead. Some of the challenges were criminal but the players would dust themselves down and go again. 'It was just the way the game was played back then,' as Leeds' Paul Madeley later remarked.

You may not have heard of the Football Act but it was passed by the Parliament of Scotland on 26 May 1424, under the reign of James I. It stated, 'The king forbiddis that na man play at the fut ball under the payne of iiij d.' In other words, football was forbidden by the monarch and punishable by a fine of four pence. Apparently this futile game called 'fut ball' was causing too many injuries and distracting the subjects when they ought to be practising something much more useful to the monarchy, like archery. Similar efforts were made in England, where Edward IV said he wanted bowmen, not ballers.

Unfortunately for James I, football refused to be outlawed, growing into the game it is today. It's still rough. It's a contact sport and so there will always be injuries – some inflicted to the head. 'You've got to look at it the correct way,' concludes Terry Butcher. 'We're talking about players' lives. We're not talking about winning games. Football becomes completely immaterial. It's secondary, miles behind what is important. In today's game it would never happen, staying on like I did, and rightfully so.' That's true in a way. Today's Laws of the Game state that a player must leave the pitch at the sight of blood. Because of that, we won't be seeing white shirts stained red on a football field any time soon, like that night in Stockholm.

And yet the modern game remains in something of a macho mess. There will be a collision, a concussion, and, so long as he can stand on two feet, an insistence from the player that he can play on. Days before this book was submitted, Leeds United's Robin Koch was left with blood pouring down his face after being blindsided by Manchester United's Scott McTominay. It was a cheap challenge; the sort synonymous with this feisty fixture. His head was wrapped in bandages, à la Terry Butcher, and he continued. Seventeen minutes later he dropped down, holding his temple and seemingly telling the bench that his vision was blurred. Only then did he walk off, gingerly and aided by an assistant. Leeds insisted they followed the Premier League's concussion protocols. Maybe so, though if that's the case, they're hardly worth the paper they're written on. Once again, football's 'never say die' nature was there for all to see, just like in Sweden in 1989.

# 11

# 'Ref, Is This the World Cup Final?'

*A concussion crisis consisting of controversies,
conflicts and protocols not fit for purpose*

'TELL HIM he's Pelé and get him back on.' It's one of football's most famous quotes and yet who said it first, if at all, remains a mystery. Partick Thistle manager John Lambie supposedly said it in response to being told that his striker Colin McGlashan was concussed and didn't know who he was. Brian Clough apparently said it about Stuart Pearce, another one-liner from the legendary boss of Nottingham Forest. Graeme Souness seemingly said it about Neil 'Razor' Ruddock after the Liverpool centre-back hurt his head while equalising against Manchester United on 4 January 1994. After trailing 3-0 inside 24 minutes, this goal made the game 3-3 and an instant Premier League classic.

Cue bedlam at Anfield. Cameras capture the Kop going berserk; a sea of limbs celebrating this late leveller. They show Jamie Redknapp screaming to the heavens. They zoom in on Liverpool's relieved-looking coaches. Meanwhile, the scorer of the goal, the man who has just saved his side from defeat to a rival, is holding his head. He's losing his balance and practically using a hug from Ian Rush to remain upright. 'Neil Ruddock,' roars Martin Tyler on the commentary, 'with a really lionhearted header.'

Replays show how, in the process of scoring, he clashed heads with Gary Pallister. According to his autobiography, *Hell Razor*, it was during the subsequent checkover that Liverpool physio Phil Boersma discovered the goalscorer didn't know who he was, where he was or what he had just done. He was Neil Ruddock, he was at Anfield, and he had scored to make it 3-3 against Manchester United, but this was news to him apparently. This message was relayed to his manager. 'At which point,' Neil wrote in *Hell Razor*, 'the quick-witted Souness quipped, "Well in that case, get back out there and tell him he's f*****g Pelé!" Sky TV wanted me to do an interview after the game but I couldn't oblige straightaway because I was too busy throwing up and nursing a wicked headache. Not that I minded too much once the lads told me what I'd done and I'd seen the goal on video later.'

Souness later said he could not recall making this off-the-cuff remark and we're unable to ask Lambie or Clough if they did as both are unfortunately no longer with us. But Neil isn't alone. Other footballers have taken hellish blows and continued, too, only to later 'wake up' at home with little recollection of how they got from A to B.

Football isn't the biggest fan of the 'C' word. It doesn't like to discuss concussion, and its authorities have never rushed to make changes which might reduce the collateral damage. The *Football Association Book for Boys* was published by English football's governing body in 1949. It was a guide for youngsters – a way of preparing any prospective talents for the realities of what it would take to be a Joe Mercer or Tommy Lawton. Flick through its pages and you'll come to a section on concussion. 'It is a common practice on the football field for an attempt to be made to restore the player by such methods as using a cold wet sponge on his face and neck, administering smelling salts, and getting him into a sitting position with his head between his knees,' it explains, alongside a sketch of a footballer being knocked backwards by a ball. 'He is then encouraged to play again as soon as possible.' First aid in football has improved since this sort of treatment, thankfully. Protocols have progressed, too, though only to an extent.

Just look at what happened on 13 July 2014. This was the day a remarkable question was asked at Rio de Janeiro's Maracanã Stadium, as reported by *La Gazzetta Dello Sport*, 'Ref, is this the final?' That is what Italian referee Nicola Rizzoli revealed he was asked by Germany's Christoph Kramer while a game of football was going on around him. It was indeed the final, and not just any final. It was Germany against Argentina in the final of the 2014 World Cup. The German had collapsed after a collision with Ezequiel Garay early on. He was treated, cleared to continue, and that's when the enquiries started with the match official. Rizzoli said, 'Shortly after the blow, Kramer came to me asking, "Ref, is this the final?" I thought he was joking and made him repeat the question and then he said, "I need to know if this is really the final." When I said "yes", he concluded, "Thanks, it was important to know that."'

The referee claimed he told Bastian Schweinsteiger about this exchange but the man with the dizzy mind remained on the pitch for 14 minutes. Clearly too groggy to continue, he was eventually substituted. The 23-year-old defensive midfielder later said something disconcerting, 'I can't remember that much from the game. I don't know anything from the first half. I thought later that I went straight off after the incident. How I got to the changing rooms, I do not know. I don't know anything else. The game, in my head, starts only in the second half.'

For this to happen on the biggest stage of them all – in a final watched by more than a billion people worldwide, according to FIFA's figures – was alarming. And yet Christoph Kramer's reputation for refusing to submit to head injuries was celebrated back home. The official YouTube channel of the Bundesliga currently boasts more than three million subscribers. On 28 November 2017, German's top tier uploaded its newest video, entitled 'Headache hero! World Cup winner Kramer knocked out again'. For your viewing pleasure, it was a highlights reel of the times the German had hurt his head but played on. 'Kramer suffered another knockout during the 2-1 win against Bayern Munchen,' read the description about the Borussia Mönchengladbach player. 'It's the third time already this season he's been struck down, and who can forget his collision during the 2014 World Cup Final in Brazil? Yet Kramer always gets back up!'

This compilation of head injuries could be considered a celebration of playing through the pain, even when concussed. The video was still available to watch on YouTube the day this book was submitted, almost five years on from its original upload. You could search 'Christoph Kramer' – as any youngsters from Mönchengladbach might – and it would have pride of place on the first page. It was a concerning message to send. The wrong message.

We've all seen those little stars circling the head of Wile E. Coyote when his pursuit of Road Runner goes wrong. He's dazed, and that's all folks. Yet it is through televised sports where children properly learn about concussion, as emphasised by a powerful two-and-a-half-minute film produced by the Concussion Legacy Foundation. Shot using a group of kids in the United States, none of them older than ten, it reminds broadcasters of the power they wield. The clip begins with each child being asked a question, 'Do you know what concussion is?' One girl shakes her head. Another shrugs her shoulders. 'Sort of,' a boy says. He is asked why certain athletes are considered tough. 'Because they had a concussion and they get back up and play.' He is asked what he would do if his coach wanted him to do that. 'I'd keep playing and try my best,' comes the reply. The film concludes by warning if your son or daughter does not know what it means to be concussed then his or her brain and future are in danger. It's a way of emphasising the need for education.

Involved in the production of this clip was Chris Nowinski. He is the former professional wrestler who was forced into early retirement, forever earning him a spot on websites listing 'five WWE superstars who retired before they turned 30'. Yet something good came out of his misery, at least. Chris, alongside Dr Robert Cantu, co-founded the Concussion Legacy Foundation. They place a particular focus on educating broadcasters so that they can educate their viewers in turn, especially the impressionable ones. 'The first time a child hears the word "concussion", it's likely to come from a sports broadcast,' Chris explains. 'We are trying to avoid situations where concussion signs and protocol breaches are ignored, which sends the message that concussions are not serious. Broadcasters need to acknowledge signs of a concussion when they occur and use the proper terminology. Describing athletes as "wobbly" or "shaking off the cobwebs" without mentioning they've likely suffered a brain injury is dangerous for children.'

Indeed, and a few too many attached to microphones have made this mistake. Fox Sports commentator Joe Buck was slated for his handling of a scary scene involving Donald Parham Jr on 16 December 2021. The Los Angeles Chargers tight end hit his head on the turf and those at home saw him lying on a stretcher, both arms shaking. 'The last thing we would ever do is speculate about any injury, especially that type,' went the Fox commentary, before indulging in some speculation. 'But when you see his arms shaking and his hands shaking on his way out, that's the part that's most unnerving. I will just add this: it is very cold, at least by Los Angeles standards.' He was later confirmed as concussed, hence the arm tremors. To combat this, the Concussion Legacy Foundation have offered complimentary training to broadcasters, including Sky Sports and BT Sport, so that their commentators know what they should and should not say.

BT have now taken up the offer and on 23 February 2022, we saw why it was needed. During their coverage of the Champions League, when Ajax's Lisandro Martinez was suspected of concussion, Michael Owen spoke dismissively of head injuries. He described them as 'bumps and bangs', adding that the reaction to these collisions was so extreme that it was as if footballers were breaking their legs. The ex-England striker was condemned for his ignorance, and it's comments like this which Chris Nowinski and co. want to keep out of the television studio.

FIFPRO, the world players' union, weren't impressed by the Christoph Kramer saga. They accused FIFA of pitiful protection during the 2014 World Cup. They said it became 'a showcase for how not to handle head injuries'. For similar incidents to occur years later at Euro 2020 emphasised the lack of progress. France's Benjamin Pavard collided with Germany's Robin Gosens in a blockbuster group game. You could see the force with which the Frenchman was pummelled and how he failed to protect his fall as he came crashing down to earth, face-planting the floor instead. 'I was a little knocked out for ten to 15 seconds,' he later said. 'After that, it was better.' This happened before the hour mark. France had not used any of their five substitutions by this stage and they didn't make their first one here. Instead the right-back, after an assessment which included water being splashed on his neck, finished the full 90.

The decision not to withdraw the player was criticised. Not least because it occurred only four days after the team doctors, head coaches and general secretaries of every nation at Euro 2020 signed a 'Concussion Charter'. That included France, who promised to substitute any man suspected of suffering from a problem. Despite this, and the player's own post-match testimony in which he said he was temporarily out cold, the competition's organisers UEFA said they were satisfied that concussion protocols were followed. Four days later, Benjamin Pavard was starting for France in their next group game against Hungary.

This was no isolated incident. At the same tournament, Austria's Christoph Baumgartner took a blow to the head in the 18th minute of their match against Ukraine. He received treatment, returned to the pitch, scored a goal in the 21st minute, then was substituted in the 33rd. 'I can't take it in yet,' the 21-year-old midfielder said afterwards. 'My skull really hurts.' When asked, UEFA said they were satisfied that protocols were followed. He started Austria's next match.

Portugal's Danilo Pereira was accidentally punched in the head by France goalkeeper Hugo Lloris, resulting in a penalty. This was in the 27th minute. The Portuguese midfielder received treatment, which included an ice pack being applied to the sensitive area, then played on. 'That's GBH,' Rio Ferdinand said in the BBC studio at half-time. 'He's whacked him in the head,' added Alan Shearer. 'Vicious,' said Gary Lineker. 'Dangerous,' said Frank Lampard. Danilo did not return for the second half. UEFA's verdict? Satisfied, again. He played Portugal's next match.

Three examples. All in the space of eight days. All at the same international tournament. All handled adequately, according to UEFA, whose most prestigious club competition has likewise courted controversy. The calamitous performance of Liverpool goalkeeper Loris Karius in the Champions League Final against Real Madrid on 26 May 2018 was linked to the fact he was concussed during the game. In the 48th minute, he was elbowed by Sergio Ramos. In the 51st he tried to roll the ball to a team-mate, only to gift a goal to Karim Benzema instead. In the 83rd he flapped at Gareth Bale's speculative strike from distance. Four days after this final, Jürgen Klopp received a phone call. It was from his friend, Franz Beckenbauer. The two-time Ballon d'Or winner had spoken to a doctor in Germany who mentioned the goalkeeper's mistakes might have been due to concussion. Interesting, he thought, so he passed the information on to Liverpool's manager. A scan was arranged at Massachusetts General Hospital in Boston where Loris was holidaying and there it was confirmed: concussion. 'Mr Karius's principal residual symptoms and objective signs suggested that visual spatial dysfunction existed and likely occurred immediately following the event,' the hospital said in a statement. 'It could be possible that such deficits would affect performance.' Yet another case of a footballer concussed on the field.

The more these incidents crop up in matches, the louder the calls for the introduction of 'temporary concussion substitutions' have grown. The idea is simple. If a footballer hurts his head, he is taken down the tunnel for a ten-minute assessment period, during which time a substitute temporarily takes his place. There is no numerical disadvantage imposed on the team, and the player benefits from a more thorough examination in private, away from prying eyes. If free from any and all symptoms of concussion at the end of this evaluation, he returns to the field. If not, the replacement stays on. It sounds simple, and it works well in other sports, such as rugby union. But then football has a habit of making the straightforward seem complex.

Wolverhampton Wanderers' Raúl Jiménez clashed heads with Arsenal's David Luiz on 29 November 2020 and landed on his side, motionless. The sound was sickening, hauntingly amplified by the Emirates Stadium's emptiness due to the Covid-19 pandemic. 'It is difficult to see your partner lifeless on the pitch,' his other half Daniela Basso later reflected in a BBC documentary called *Raúl Jiménez: Code Red*. 'Code Red' referred to what Nuno Espírito Santo, the Wolves manager at the time, heard while his striker was being strapped to a stretcher to be taken to St Mary's Hospital in London for surgery. It turned out that Raul had fractured his skull.

Worryingly, David Luiz continued, blood leaking through the bandage wrapped around his head. The collision occurred in the fifth minute of this match but it wasn't until half-time that the Brazilian centre-back was substituted. Petr Čech found that astonishing. He is the former Chelsea goalkeeper who fractured his skull after crashing into the knee of Reading's Stephen Hunt at the Madejski Stadium on 14 October 2006. For the rest of his career, he wore a protective helmet, a constant reminder of that dark day. Petr told me it was disturbing to see his old team-mate involved in a clash which resulted in the cracking of a skull and yet play on. He said this showed why temporary substitutions are a must.

Petr explained, 'Someone comes in, Luiz leaves, does the test. If he fails, he stays in the dressing room. If he's fit, then the manager has the choice. Football is a contact sport. If you take away the contact, the energy, the tackles, the physicality, then it would not be the same. But we can improve the way that injuries are dealt with. To have a substitute would take away the pressure to get the player back on the pitch. I was concussed a few times. My concussion always had a delayed effect. There was a game against Fulham in the League Cup in 2011. I collided with a player.'

The opponent was Orlando Sá and Petr can remember his head jerking backwards, as if he were a boxer who had just taken a right hook. He felt fine at first and passed the customary checks. Then at half-time, his vision blurred. He was taken to hospital where he was confirmed with concussion. 'Sometimes the doctor has limited time and for the first three or four minutes, the player is fine,' continued the man with two metal plates fitted into his skull and who is now technical and performance advisor for Chelsea. 'No symptoms. That's why the player stays on. But he can get worse. That's the problem. The substitute takes that away.' It was at this point of the conversation that Petr paused, thinking back to the day he almost died on the football field. 'It's unfortunate that you always wait for a tragedy to change rules,' he adds.

The International Football Association Board are the game's lawmakers and their Concussion Expert Group have shown a preference for 'additional permanent concussion substitutions' – the scenario where a coach can use an extra replacement in the event of a head injury, even if he's already used up his usual allocation. It has its critics, however, and so do the CEG. They consist of a mix of members. There's a former manager in Arsène Wenger, a former referee in Pierluigi Collina, and senior figures from several governing bodies. For this reason, they've been accused of being stacked with football insiders rather than brain injury specialists. It was at a meeting on 21 October 2020 that this group recommended trials. Not of temporary substitutions, but the alternative. They wanted to see whether additional permanent substitutions would work. The CEG's reasoning was this option could be implemented across all of football – not that this stopped the game from introducing VAR and goal-line technology at the highest level – and that it best reflected the 'if in doubt, sit them out' philosophy. For this, they needed guinea pigs and the Premier League put its hand up, sanctioning its use in the 2020/21 and 2021/22 seasons. It would also be trialled in the FA Cup, Women's Super League and Women's Championship.

One problem remained with these new protocols – club medics were operating under the same constraints as previously. They were waiting to be invited on to the pitch. They were providing an assessment there and then and in front of thousands of fans – millions, if you include the television audience. They were holding up a game being broadcasted globally and the cameras were filling the dead air by focusing on the player with the potential brain injury. Meanwhile, the clock on that scoreboard was tick, tick, ticking away. Colin Lewin, the former physiotherapist for Arsenal, described this pressure as a 'privilege' when asked about it, 'The first few games you're the pitch physio, you're a little apprehensive, you're desperate to get things right, you're making sure everything is in place. But when you get to the 500th game, it's back to the training. It becomes routine.' There is no suggestion that team doctors do not have the players' health at heart. They're medical professionals whose oath is to protect their patient, first and foremost. But they are, and always have been, thrown into silly situations by the parameters within which they must work.

The history books will forever show that West Ham United's Issa Diop was English football's first concussion substitute. It was in an FA Cup fifth-round match against Manchester United at Old Trafford on 9 February 2021. This was three days after the trial's official start date and it was criticised for failing its very first test. The West Ham centre-back had dropped down in the 37th minute following a clash of heads and he wasn't substituted until half-time. 'The decision to allow Diop to return to the field of play after being assessed for concussion in just two minutes, while still on the pitch, shows just how deeply flawed this new protocol is,' said Peter McCabe, the chief executive of Headway, the brain injury charity. This example was cited in a letter to IFAB, sent from the players' union PFA and world players' union FIFPRO, on 14 April 2021. They weren't blaming the club medics. They were blaming the pathetic protocols. It was time to trial temporary substitutions instead, they said, adding a poll of 96 doctors from English, Belgian and French clubs found 83 per cent preferred this option.

When a Premier League player is concussed, he can return to playing by the following week. Critics say that's convenient for the product but not the participants. The Football Association's return-to-play protocols involve six stages, each of which can be completed in 24 hours, starting with 'initial rest period' and ending with 'return to play'. Suddenly the footballer who suffered that brain injury on Saturday is at stage six and back in time for the following game. Numerous studies have suggested a one-week turnaround is nowhere near adequate, however. Some even say the effects of concussion can last as long as 30 days. And yet footballers can only trust that for all their qualifications, those who set this timeframe on their behalf know best. It brings to mind the scene in *Monty Python's The Meaning of Life* in which a mother is giving birth. 'What do I do?' she asks. 'Nothing, dear,' responds the doctor played by John Cleese. 'You're not qualified!'

Look closely at the fine print of the FA's concussion protocols and you'll see the inspiration. 'The guidelines,' declares the document, 'are in line with the Consensus Statement on Concussion in Sport issued by the Fifth International Conference on Concussion in Sport, Berlin 2016.' You may not have heard of the Concussion in Sport Group behind this conference, but they're an important bunch. Every four years, the CISG meet to review the latest research and at the end of this symposium, an assembly of around 40 experts produce a consensus statement – a document described as the 'bible' of concussion guidelines as it provides an overview of the latest knowledge. It is the most influential medical paper of its kind produced because of its sway in sport worldwide, from youth to adult, amateur to professional. If you're a footballer who's had concussion, it's probable you were diagnosed using the SCAT5 or CRT5, both of which are recommended by the CISG for sideline assessments. If you're a fan wondering why your player is unavailable – like how Liverpool's Curtis Jones missed the start of the 2021/22 season – it's because, as previously stated, the FA are among the many organisations who base their protocols on this consensus statement.

It was at the Ritz-Carlton Hotel in Berlin on 27 October 2016 that the CISG gathered for the start of the latest conference. One of the attendees was Professor Jiří Dvořák, chief medical officer of world governing body FIFA. Outlining their influence, he estimated they were representing 'one billion professional and amateur athletes' in football, ice hockey, equestrian and rugby alone. Prof Dvořák has attended every conference since the CISG's first in Zurich in 2001. The consensus statement published at the conclusion of Berlin 2016 would shape policies in sport for longer than expected due to the Covid-19 pandemic. The CISG's next rendezvous was supposed to be held in Paris in 2020 but it was postponed, and so was the 2021 conference.

Had they managed to meet at the Marriott Rive Gauche Hotel as planned, they would have devised protocols which would impact Paris Saint-Germain's horde of superstars at the Parc des Princes, a 20-minute drive from the Marriott. And every club in England. And Spain. And Italy. Everywhere, really. This was another sorry consequence of Covid – no conference and so no updated guide on how to deal with concussion. It was rescheduled, again, for Amsterdam in 2022.

As the CISG's work is so important, their power is scrutinised. Rightly so, too. On 19 October 2021, a group of 17 researchers, clinicians and caregivers released a paper calling for a radical revamp of a process they branded 'narrow, compromised and flawed'. Entitled 'Toward Complete, Candid, and Unbiased International Consensus Statements on Concussion in Sport', they attacked the CISG. They accused them of promoting 'sports-friendly' protocols rather than taking a 'precautionary, public health and patient-centred' stance. They criticised them for not inviting those 'who have paid, or are paying, the high price that repeated exposure to concussion in sports can exact' to be part of the process, such as the mother who lost a son, wife who lost a husband, or former footballer who fears losing his mind. They insisted it was wrong that these Consensus Statements were instead 'dominated by individuals with close relationships' to sports organisations, saying such 'potential conflicts' should be explicitly signposted. In short, they said it was time for an overhaul.

It is true that the CISG is sponsored by sporting bodies, such as the International Olympic Committee, World Rugby and FIFA, and the signatories themselves can have past or present connections to organisations. An analysis by Canada's CBC News looked at the résumés of the 36 panellists involved in the last statement, reporting 32 had ties to corporations. Prof Dvořák was one of those named and he defended the impartiality of their work when I contacted him. He insisted there was no influence from their benefactors, adding that his personal involvement with FIFA ended in 2016. 'The CISG works independently from any institution,' he said while claiming it's no closed shop and that there are plenty involved without ties to the sponsoring bodies. Naturally, though, the connections which do exist concern outsiders who say it's all too closely intertwined for their liking. If anyone disagrees with the consensus on the day, they can file a dissenting opinion or withdraw their name from authorship. No one privileged enough to be inside the Ritz-Carlton in 2016 staged such a protest.

There were plenty on the outside who did voice their disapproval upon reading the CISG's report, however. Not least when it came to their position on Chronic Traumatic Encephalopathy. 'The notion that repeated concussion or subconcussive impacts cause CTE remains unknown,' they decided. With CTE only being identified in American football relatively recently, the science is young and so the spectrum of opinion is wide. Yet this was a conservative viewpoint, to say the least.

In coming to this verdict, the CISG reviewed all available research on the long-term repercussions of sports-related concussion. There was plenty to pore over. Yet of the 3,819 studies identified, only 47 were deemed worthy of inclusion, thanks to the high standard set by their criteria. One of the 15 authors involved in this systematic review was Christopher Randolph, who's never sat on the fence with CTE. In 2014 he wrote an article asking whether it was a verifiable condition, entitled 'Is Chronic Traumatic Encephalopathy a real disease?' In 2018, he concluded it wasn't, writing another called 'Chronic Traumatic Encephalopathy is not a real disease'. Another author was Professor Paul McCrory, who gained a reputation as a chief cheerleader in denying CTE is connected to repetitive head trauma. You only need to note his description of the noise in the NFL – calling it 'all the carry on and hoo-ha you get from the United States' – to understand his stance. He uttered those words at a lecture called 'The Concussion "Crisis" – Media, Myths and Medicine' in which he suggested the press make too much of head injuries in sports like American football. You can watch a video of that talk on YouTube today. Find it on The Florey Institute of Neuroscience and Mental Health's channel and decide for yourself whether you find it as patronising as I did upon first viewing.

Of the five Consensus Statements to date, Prof McCrory was lead author of four of them. Another with past ties to sporting bodies, his was a position of influence. His fingerprints were all over the literature on traumatic brain injuries and this concussion kingpin was all set to chair Amsterdam 2022. That was until he faced accusations of plagiarism – the practice that is considered a cardinal sin in academia, up there with faking data. After it was alleged that he'd been passing off others' work as his own, Prof McCrory offered his resignation. The CISG accepted it, though perhaps failed to read the room when releasing a statement praising their colleague's 'significant clinical and research contribution to the field of concussion in sport over more than two decades'.

A community of athletes trusted the CISG to have their best interests at heart but this risked tainting their reputation. Suddenly sporting bodies were reviewing their relationship with – and reliance on – this besieged group. That included FIFA, one of their beneficiaries, and those calls for an overhaul were as loud as they had ever been when this book was sent to print. Prof McCrory's work was under scrutiny, including the leading part he played in those Consensus Statements which were criticised for failing to recommend the strictest concussion protocols and downplaying CTE.

Prof McCrory's departure was celebrated by plenty, given their perception of him as a bad apple. But then what about the rest of the fruit basket who willingly put their name to this document?

The idea that CTE is fake news doesn't wash with the wives and widows of former footballers who insist they witnessed the tell-tale signs of the disease develop in their beau. Their qualifications for this claim? They lived with it. Day in, day out. In the same household, in the same bed. To them, denial is disrespect. They fear today's players remain at risk of the toxic tau protein spreading through their brains like poison ivy so long as they're subjected to concussion and subconcussion. That is partly why they take that difficult decision to donate to science – to prove to themselves, to the deniers, to all of football that this problem exists. Five years on from Berlin 2016, in the week that Paris 2021 should have been taking place, I was curious as to whether the attitude towards CTE had changed. Speaking anonymously to one attendee of that conference in the German capital, the disease was described as 'science fiction', 'flimsy', a 'false narrative', a 'theory', a 'hypothesis' and a 'finding under a microscope' over the course of our conversation. By no means were these comments made on behalf of the CISG, who would have another six years of research to review come Amsterdam 2022. But it was a curious insight into how CTE continues to divide the scientific community with some still insistent that there's nothing to see here.

Despite its naysayers, there is no denying that these three little letters are now known to the common person, nowhere more so than in the United States. Fans of American football can watch the Hollywood film *Concussion*, starring Will Smith as Dr Bennet Omalu, the pathologist who first discovered the disease in four-time Super Bowl winner Mike Webster. They can browse the Wikipedia page listing the NFL players confirmed with CTE. They can check the concussion settlement website to see whether payments have passed the billion-dollar mark. At the time of writing, the total stood at $963m, though it should be noted that this arrangement did not represent an admission of guilt by the NFL, who maintain they did no wrong. The CISG may not have been entirely convinced by CTE or what causes it at Berlin 2016, citing a need for further research. But then campaigners say there are a billion reasons why it should be of concern right now.

The war of words will continue. One side will say they do good work, and the other will say it's nowhere near good enough. Yet it is important to remember those stuck in the middle of this mess and that's the sportsmen and women in the midst of a concussion crisis. They're the ones being treated for brain injuries in front of thousands of supporters. They're the ones having their onboard computers temporarily taken offline, only to be told they've rebooted and are good to go by the following weekend. They're the ones asking if they're playing in a World Cup final.

# 12

# The Boys of '66

*Once champions of the world, England's 1966
heroes have been decimated by dementia*

IF YOU received a letter from the Football Association on 10
May 1966, it meant you were going to Lilleshall for a two-week
training camp. 'As you will have read in the press you have been
selected for the World Cup training party,' it opened. Imagine
the rush. The shivers. The frantic thoughts of what to pack
and where to be and when. It was not only mailed to the 28
players but staff members, too. Among the recipients was Dr
Neil Phillips, an invitation to act as England team doctor. He
was to deputise for regular medical man Dr Alan Bass, who was
unavailable between 6 and 17 June due to work commitments at
St Mary's Hospital in London. Dr Phillips agreed to substitute
and arrived at Lilleshall with two orders – to weigh the players
daily and inspect their feet. However, he was also surprised as,
upon rocking up, he discovered there were no medical supplies.
Not even a roll of Elastoplast, as Dr Phillips later recounted in
his book *Doctor To The World Champions*. All he had on him was
his personal bag – the one he used as a GP in Redcar.

As a teenager, Dr Phillips had taken a foot to the head while
playing rugby and fractured his skull. What can happen when
sport goes wrong was imprinted in his brain in more ways than
one. He knew the risks. Yet his first morning in charge of the

England squad was spent at the local chemist's store, no doubt making the shopkeeper's day as he bought the bulk of his stock. It is a little-known story, a light-hearted tale, and one which makes Sir Geoff Hurst laugh when I remind him of it. 'That really sums it up,' says the former centre-forward whose three goals turned England into world champions. 'The difference between then and now; between playing in the medieval days and the modern day.'

Sir Geoff concedes he is somewhat lucky. Why he retained his mental faculties while his friends lost theirs, he cannot say. Of the England team that immortalised themselves on 30 July 1966 at Wembley, defeating West Germany 4-2 in extra time, five men have disclosed their dementia diagnoses to the world – Ray Wilson, Martin Peters, Jack Charlton, Nobby Stiles and Sir Bobby Charlton. The manager, Sir Alf Ramsey, had the disease, too. Because of this, England's greatest team risks being remembered for the wrong reasons. We would love it if the legacy of 1966 was merely one of joy. Of a band of brothers coming together to win at Wembley. Of Bobby Moore sitting on his team-mates' shoulders. Of Nobby dancing with the Jules Rimet Trophy in one hand and his dentures in the other. Of Kenneth Wolstenholme announcing, 'People are on the pitch, they think it's all over; it is now.' Yet it is with great sadness that this final, this victory, this team have also come to symbolise something much darker – the fragility of the footballer's brain.

The plight of England's 1966 World Cup winners prompted the *Mail on Sunday* to wonder whether this disturbingly high rate of diagnosis extended to the domestic game. To find out, they performed an 'audit' of the preceding season, which would conclude with English football's finest summer. First they researched the squads of the 1965/66 season, leaving them with a pool of 475 players at the 22 First Division clubs. The *Mail's* Nick Harris, James Sharpe and Cara Sloman then worked their way through that list, one by one. Whether they died and of what cause. Whether they were alive and well. Whether they were living with dementia. They checked records, contacted clubs, asked associations and spoke with families. 'In many cases we were being told, off the record, that a living player had dementia but it wasn't public,' Nick recalls.

This process took the three of them several weeks, until finally, on 22 November 2020, they were ready to reveal their findings. They found neurodegenerative disease was a factor in 42 per cent of the deaths of top-flight footballers who played in 1965/66. Of the 475 players, 185 had died at the time of this report, and at least 79 of those were connected to conditions associated with traumatic brain injury. The average age of death was 74. So it wasn't some anomaly that half of England's 1966 World Cup winners were diagnosed with dementia. It was entirely fitting.

The England players didn't practise much heading at Lilleshall in truth. Most of that happened at club level. 'At West Ham, we had a ball hanging in the gym,' explains Sir Geoff. 'It was a long swinging ball, from as high as 20ft, coming down from the ceiling. So you had that practice, then we'd play head tennis together, then you had the practice on the pitch. We were well-known at West Ham for creating goals at the near post, that cross and header.' Just look at the winner against Argentina in the World Cup quarter-final on 23 July 1966. A Martin Peters cross and a Sir Geoff Hurst header – a goal made by West Ham. 'That was all honed on the training ground,' Sir Geoff says. At Lilleshall, however, Sir Alf placed a greater focus on fitness. England's manager told his team in a meeting they may not be the most talented bunch to grace the tournament, but by gum, they would be the fittest. So they ran, and ran, and ran some more.

In a warm-up friendly against Denmark on 3 July, Sir Geoff didn't give the greatest account of himself. He blames the training session the day before which left him leggy. He didn't start the World Cup opener, a 0-0 stalemate with Uruguay. Or the game after that, a 2-0 win over Mexico. Or the game after that, another 2-0 victory over France. Yet he replaced Jimmy Greaves for the quarter-final against Argentina, the semi-final against Portugal and then the final against West Germany, scoring a perfect hat-trick – right foot, left foot, header. 'It's not a day you forget,' he tells me. For a handful of his old team-mates, though, it was. This day of English delight and German grief became a blur in their minds.

Imagine the celebrations today if England won the World Cup. The parties. The parades. The frothy mist from the plastic pint glasses flying through the air. After leaving Wembley in 1966, England's players retreated to the Royal Garden Hotel in Kensington for a champagne dinner in the presence of prime minister Harold Wilson. Outside, supporters congregated to congratulate the boys. It was described as being 'like VE night, election night and New Year's Eve rolled into one'. Inside, the team enjoyed a dignified evening together, occasionally removing themselves from the banqueting hall to appear on the balcony with the Jules Rimet Trophy. They were officially the Boys of '66, and they never lost their appetite for an evening in each others' company.

Years later these World Cup winners would cross paths on the after-dinner circuit. Jack Charlton joked at one such function that his plans for a summer of fishing and shooting had been ruined. The reason was the Republic of Ireland, the team he was managing, had made it to the 1994 World Cup. 'Qualifying has buggered my summer up!' He was a good-humoured man, Big Jack, and his team-mates enjoyed these fleeting encounters.

Soon enough, these champions started wondering why they only waited for these black tie events to meet. Why catch up in front of an audience? Why not organise a gathering of our own?

So they did. The winners and the wives, a golf getaway and good times. It became an annual affair and they took it in turns to host these weekend jaunts. The 2013 edition was organised by Wolverhampton Wanderers legend and 1966 squad member Ron Flowers, for example, and took place at Brocton Hall Golf Club. A round or two, a pint or three, and plenty of reminiscing about *that* day at Wembley. Both Charlton brothers were there, along with Nobby Stiles, Gordon Banks, Roger Hunt and more. Sadly this would be one of their final get-togethers as a group. The yearly event had lasted for two decades before numbers started to dwindle.

Ray Wilson was the first of the diagnosed players to pass away, aged 83 on 15 May 2018. He was the left-back who liked to stay out of the limelight but remained a regular at Huddersfield Town games despite his dementia diagnosis in 2004. Martin Peters followed at the age of 76 on 21 December 2019. He was the midfielder who, concerned about muddying the Queen's white gloves, made sure to rid his right hand of any dirt on his way up to Wembley's Royal Box. His loved ones say that was entirely in keeping with his character. Always thinking of others. Even after winning the World Cup, it seems. Martin's wife, Kathleen, spoke with Judith Hurst daily for decades. 'Every single day,' says Sir Geoff. Though the Hurst family were not cursed by dementia directly, they were as close as can be to someone who was.

Jack Charlton was the next to depart, aged 85 on 10 July 2020. The wonderful documentary *Finding Jack Charlton* offers an intimate insight into the man and the final 18 months of his life. The original plan was to tell the story of an Englishman becoming an honorary Irishman. Of beating England at Euro 1988. Of back-to-back World Cups. Of a national team transformed. Yet Jack's dementia was too advanced to allow him to discuss his days managing the Republic of Ireland. We see that on screen. 'They think a lot of you, don't they, in Ireland?' asks Pat, Jack's wife. 'I have no idea,' he answers. So the documentary evolved to not only focus on the good old days but also the difficult new ones. While watching grainy footage of himself from a 1980 travelogue *The Coast of King Jack*, he sits back. 'That's me,' he tells his family of the lanky figure wearing beige flares and walking by Dunstanburgh Castle. 'I don't even know [it's] me doing it,' he adds. Another scene shows Jack sitting at his kitchen table. This time he's being shown footage of himself stood in front of the Ireland squad the night they were knocked out of the 1990 World Cup by hosts Italy. 'Ohhhh me lads, you shudda seen us gannin'.' Forever proud of his north-east roots, he's singing that classic Geordie ballad 'Blaydon Races'. Only he knows the words. Only he needs to know them. All Irish eyes are on the Englishman in the white short-sleeved shirt and black tie singing on this balmy summer's night in Rome. Pat asks her husband if he can remember serenading his players and staff. Jack says nothing. Her right hand on his left shoulder offering reassurance, she says it will come flooding back the next time he watches it. 'Yes, probably,' comes the reply.

It is in these moments that this much-loved football man's fogginess is laid bare. Yet filmmakers did not want *Finding Jack Charlton* to centre on pity. 'When we filmed with Jack, we did scenes where he was still with his charity, still with his grandkids, still fishing, still active,' says Gabriel Clarke, who directed the documentary with Pete Thomas. 'He was still aware of the camera. In fact he liked the camera. As his son says in the film, "Good days and bad days." You can continue to live a life. That was really important for us.' And for the family. They did not want dementia to define this husband, father and grandfather. To the very end, Jack was living life as well as he could, still wearing a smile and that flat cap of his.

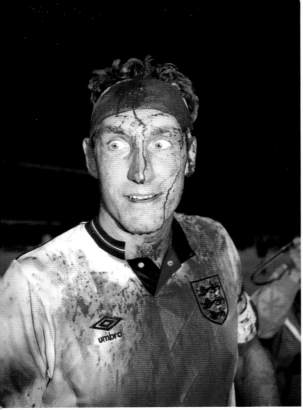

Terry Butcher's white England shirt is stained red after completing their World Cup qualifier against Sweden with an open head wound in September 1989 – a decision he later described as 'foolish'

West Bromwich Albion striker Jeff Astle celebrates scoring the winner against Everton in the 1968 FA Cup Final at Wembley Stadium.

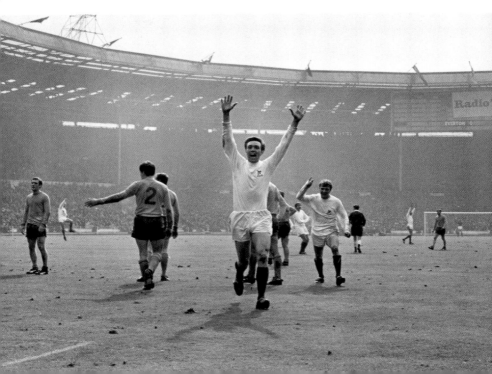

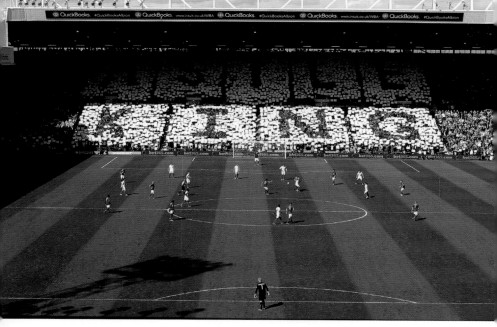

Supporters spell 'ASTLE KING' while the players wear a one-off replica strip from the 1968 FA Cup Final in honour of their former striker who died with dementia.

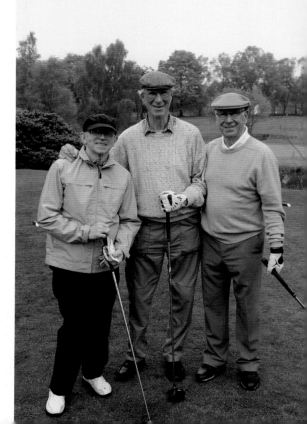

Nobby Stiles, Jack Charlton and Sir Bobby Charlton at Brocton Hall Golf Club in May 2013. All three 1966 World Cup winners developed dementia.

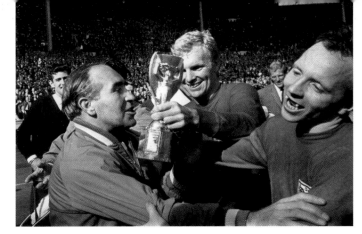

*England manager Sir Alf Ramsey kisses the Jules Rimet trophy with captain Bobby Moore and Nobby Stiles.*

*Chris Sutton poses with his dad, Mike, who played professionally and died with dementia, after signing for Blackburn Rovers for £5m in 1994.*

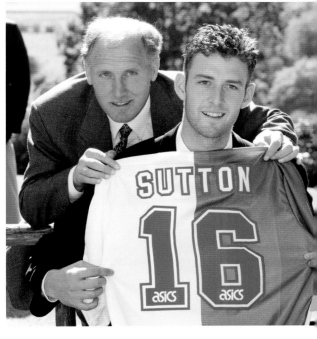

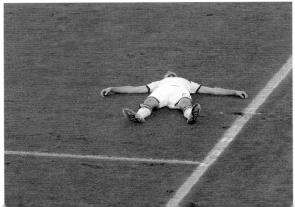

*Germany's Christoph Kramer lies on the pitch after a collision during the 2014 World Cup Final against Argentina. He played on and Italian official Nicola Rizzoli later revealed he asked him, 'Ref, is this the final?'*

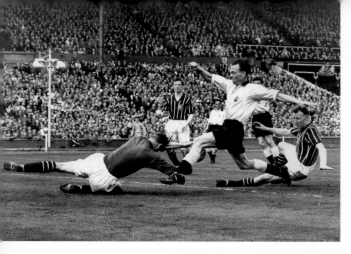

*Manchester City goalkeeper Bert Trautmann dives at the feet of Birmingham City's Peter Murphy during the 1956 FA Cup Final. It was whilst making this save that he broke his neck before playing on.*

*Dr Bennet Omalu with Will Smith, who played him in the Hollywood film* Concussion *about the discovery of CTE in the NFL.*

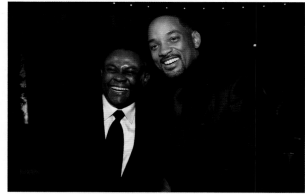

*Dr Ann McKee stands over the brain of an unnamed former NFL player. She is the director of Boston University's CTE Centre and its Brain Bank.*

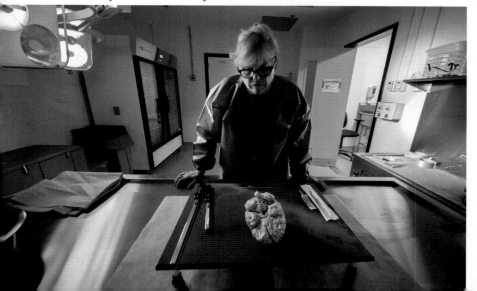

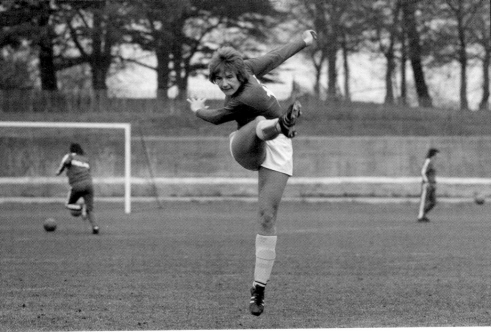

*Sue Lopez after taking a shot in training for England in November 1974. Sue became the first female player to publicly link her dementia to her career.*

*Arsenal's David Luiz continues to play with blood leaking from his bandages after a clash of heads with Wolverhampton Wanderers' Raul Jimenez, who fractured his skull in the collision in November 2020.*

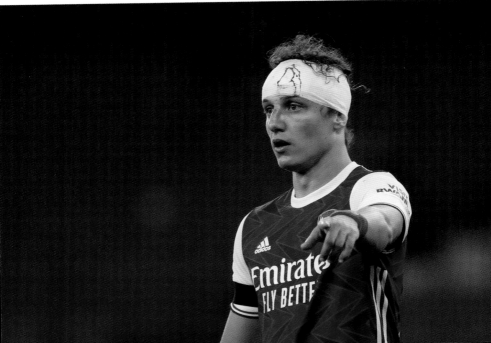

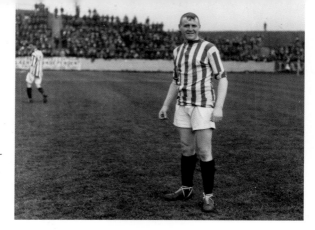

Manchester United captain Charlie Roberts in September 1912. Charlie set up the players' union, today known as the PFA, and went on to die after a seven-and-a-half-hour operation on his brain.

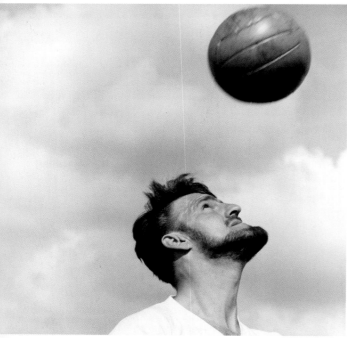

Jimmy Hill heads a ball in August 1960. Jimmy developed dementia and it's been claimed one of his former clubs would soak the leather ball in a bucket of water overnight to make it gain weight.

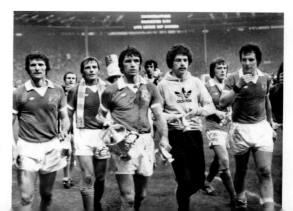

Dave Watson walks with the 1976 League Cup trophy and has blood dripping down his Manchester City shirt after a clash of heads. Dave, described as 'the forgotten England captain' by his wife, Penny, now has dementia.

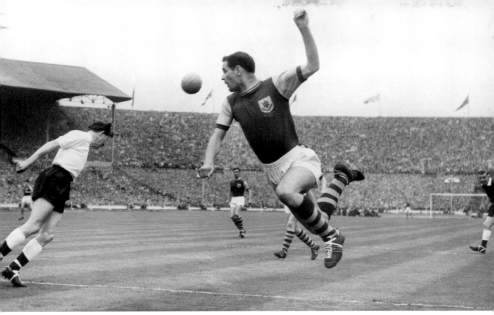

*Burnley's Jimmy Robson after jumping to meet a cross in the 1962 FA Cup Final as Tottenham Hotspur's Danny Blanchflower heads clear. Both men developed dementia later in life.*

*Seven of Burnley's 1959/60 title-winning team developed dementia, indicated in bold. Top row, left to right: Alex Elder,* **Jimmy Robson**, **Tommy Cummings**, **Adam Blacklaw**, *Brian Miller, John Angus,* **Ray Pointer**. *Front row, left to right: John Connelly,* **Jimmy McIlroy**, **Jimmy Adamson**, **Brian Pilkington**, *Trevor Meredith.*

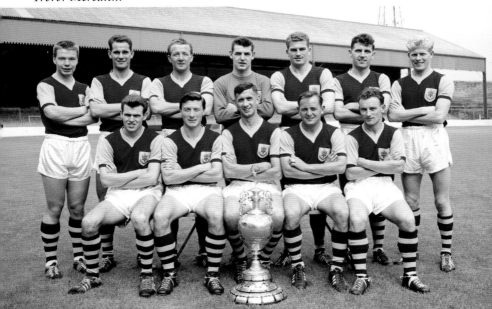

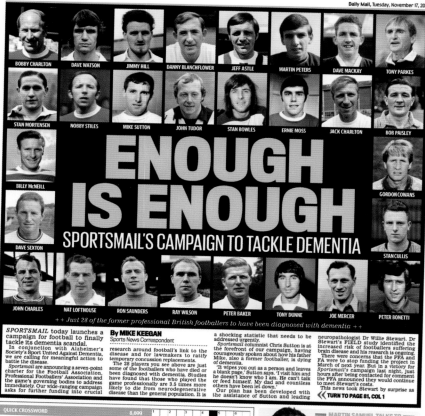

The back page of the Daily Mail on 17 November 2020 showing just 28 of the former British footballers diagnosed with dementia.

The article which appeared in FIFA Magazine – the world governing body's own publication – in 1984 warning of the dangers of heading the ball.

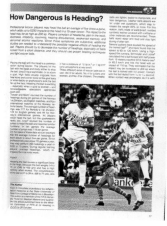

The documentary's most raw scene, the one which moved me to tears, was saved for last. Jack is on his own, sitting and staring ahead. A record is spinning on a turntable in front of him. It's playing 'Blaydon Races'. Then comes the chorus, and suddenly the arms of Jack are outstretched, those big fists clenched. Fog? What fog? All is clear now. Jack remembers and just like 30 years ago, he's singing along to his favourite anthem. 'Ohhhh me lads, you shudda seen us gannin', passin' the folks alang the road jus' as they wor stannin', there was lotsa lads an' lasses there, all wi' smiling faces, gannin' alang the Scotswood Rooooad, to see the Blaydon Races.' The final shot is a close-up of Jack's eyes, as piercing blue as they always were.

It should be noted that Jack's family do not blame football. Pat says she isn't sure what caused her husband to develop dementia. His son, John, doesn't believe it was down to heading the ball. The game gave Jack a great life. This boy from the coal-mining village of Ashington lived the dream as a player. As a manager he delighted in opponents knowing the secrets of his Ireland team's style of play, because he figured there was 'bugger all' they could do about it. That was Jack – beautifully straightforward and original. When *Finding Jack Charlton* premiered, it concluded a week-long campaign to raise money for The Alzheimer Society of Ireland. More than €1m was made, such was the love for Big Jack among the Irish audience.

It was on 30 October 2020 that Nobby Stiles died at the age of 78. There was no one in football like Nobby. There's never been anyone like him since. In his own words, he was the 'weedy-looking, short-sighted, 5ft 5½in bloke with a top plate of false teeth'. Not your typical sporting hero, but that's what he became. He wasn't always so admired, mind. Whereas the midfield destroyers of today can be celebrated, Nobby wasn't the most popular of players. He was all too aware of that. Before the World Cup, as a Manchester United player, he received a letter with a Liverpool postmark. 'Dear Ugly,' it read. 'Don't look round when you come down the tunnel on Saturday because you might get a hatchet in your head.' During the World Cup, after a particularly robust challenge wiped out French playmaker Jacques Simon in England's final group game, he was vilified. The son of an undertaker from Collyhurst, Manchester, it was written in France that he was the greatest advertisement for his father's business. Danny Blanchflower, working for the BBC, said it ruined the game. FIFA decided it was 'rough play' and issued a retrospective yellow card after referee Arturo Yamasaki had missed the foul in real time. There was even a campaign to get 'nasty Nobby' out of the England team for being the lion who roars too loud.

Good job the manager took no notice of this nonsense. On 22 July 1966, the England team were at Highbury, the home of Arsenal, practising free kicks and corners. The next day they would be facing Argentina in an all-or-nothing quarter-final. 'Did you mean it?' Sir Alf Ramsey had approached his toothless terrier and wanted to know the truth. 'No, Alf, I didn't,' said Nobby. He explained the quick-thinking Frenchman had merely moved the ball a split second before his arrival. 'You're playing tomorrow,' the manager said. And that was it. 'My dad was over the moon,' Nobby's son, John, says. 'He was certain he was going to be left out. Ramsey was then summoned up to the boardroom at Highbury and told, in no uncertain terms, that Stiles should not play tomorrow. Ramsey told his bosses that if he didn't play against Argentina then they could find themselves a new manager. He threatened to resign.'

Despite kicking lumps out of each other, Leeds United and Scotland hard man Billy Bremner sent Nobby a telegram. 'Keep your chin up,' it read. But Nobby couldn't help worrying. 'The next morning, my dad is on the coach on the way to Wembley, thinking the whole country is against him. He's sat next to Bally

– Alan Ball – who nudges him and says, "Look at that."' Out of the window, in a north London street, was a banner surrounded by around 100 supporters. 'Nobby for Prime Minister' it read. Suddenly he felt ten feet tall and once at Wembley, he went through his usual process.

They were a superstitious lot, the England team of 1966. Gordon Banks had to shake every player's hand. Jack Charlton had to be the last out of the changing room. Then there was Nobby. Poached egg on toast his pre-match meal. Cup of tea his tipple. Always tied his laces out on the field. Never shaved until two hours before kick off. Teeth out. Glasses off. Contacts in. For all six matches, he rocked up at Wembley wearing the same suit, same shirt, same tie, vest, socks and cufflinks. Any deviation and he would feel lousy. Nobby was concerned prior to the semi-final against Portugal, for example, because his dry-cleaning was not ready at the team's Hendon Hall Hotel. Thankfully he got his outfit back in time then he proceeded to place Eusébio in his pocket. Ahead of facing Argentina, while organising himself, two visitors risked upsetting his routine but they felt it was necessary. One was England assistant Harold Shepherdson. 'Don't you let Alf down,' he said. 'He's gone to bat for you.' The other was coach Les Cocker. 'Don't let Alf down,' he added.

Nobby didn't. He wasn't the most popular player before the World Cup, and definitely not during. But afterwards, he was the new darling of the nation. 'The whole thing turned,' says John, who also played football professionally. Nobby, whose team-mates' nickname for him was 'Happy', acknowledged his newfound popularity in a column for the *Sunday Mirror* three weeks after his toothless jig at Wembley. 'I feel a hero,' he wrote. 'I've been made one by the World Cup.'

As a distributor of blows, Nobby absorbed his fair share on the field, too. He also headed the ball. Not so much in matches, but he practised it as much as the next man. 'My dad played in the back four at Manchester United,' John says. 'Him and Bill Foulkes were having balls fired at them in training.' His memory first started to fail him at age 60 but he continued to work. For years, Nobby and John travelled the country together, a father and son double act. 'He was a speaker. I was a comedian. It was brilliant. Then in 2013, he had a big dip. This is what I've found with footballers. They lose their memory, and lose their memory, and lose their memory, then they have a big dip. Anxiety takes over. Paranoia. They can't be on their own. After that happened, we never really got him back.'

Nobby's family donated his brain to Professor Willie Stewart. 'If by donating his brain, we can stop one person from suffering the way your dad did, then we'll do it,' decided his widow, Kay. The results confirmed the family's fears. 'He didn't have Alzheimer's,' says John, who apologises for choking up while discussing his dad. 'It was CTE that his brain was riddled with. When the results came through, it was validation and an awful lot of anger. I was raging. They've known about this since the 1960s. When my dad was dying in his home, my mum was still getting letters asking him to attend Football Association functions for free.'

Football wasn't awash with money back then. Winning the World Cup did not make these men immediate millionaires. They fulfilled hearts but not their bank accounts. The original plan was that every England player in the 22-man squad would receive a £500 bonus, with additional appearance money for those who actually played. Captain Bobby Moore wasn't happy with that arrangement. 'No,' he said, standing up during a meeting. 'We're a squad. We stick together.' He demanded each player received £1,000, regardless of whether he appeared in all six matches or none at all. 'I thought you might say that, Robert,' Sir Alf is said to have replied to his skipper with a smile.

Later in life, many of these men resorted to selling their medals, including Nobby. An auction of his memorabilia in Edinburgh in 2010 raised £424,438, with Manchester United paying more than £200,000 for his World Cup and European Cup winners' medals. Some needed funds to cover rising care costs. Others wanted to leave something behind for their families. They sold prized possessions, spoke after dinners, signed books, appeared on television shows, flogged Carlsberg lager and Shredded Wheat cereal and Marks & Spencer suits.

Sir Bobby Charlton was unable to attend the service for Nobby. The week before, Lady Norma announced her husband was the fifth member of England's World Cup winners diagnosed with dementia. It featured on every newspaper's back page – and several front pages – on 2 November 2020. This was *the* man of English football and the country's greatest-ever sportsman in the estimations of some. He survived the Munich air disaster which stole the lives of 23 people, including eight Manchester United players, on 6 February 1958, then was pictured sitting in a hospital bed with bandages wrapped around his head. It was remarkable that he returned to playing less than a month later, appearing in the FA Cup quarter-final against West Bromwich Albion on 1 March. He was 20 years old.

Sir Bobby delivered for club and country. He won the 1968 European Cup, scoring twice in the final against Benfica. He won the 1966 World Cup, scoring twice in the semi-final against Portugal. What Sir Bobby can recall of these majestic matches, only he and his family know, though this 1966 Ballon d'Or winner's legacy will never be lost.

You may not recognise the name, but Tommy Charlton is the younger brother of Sir Bobby and Jack. Just like his siblings, he too represented his country. Sir Bobby made his England debut on 19 April 1958, aged 20 in a 4-0 win over Scotland at Hampden Park. Jack on 10 April 1965, aged 29, appeared in a

2-2 draw with Scotland at Wembley. Tommy made his debut on 13 May 2018, at the age of 71. It was for England's over-60s in the first-ever walking football international tournament. Wearing the iconic red, England beat Italy 3-0 at Brighton's Amex Stadium to take the trophy. Before the game, Tommy received a message from Jack. It made him emotional then, and it makes him emotional now as he recounts it, 'Hope you have a good game. Thinking of you. Sorry we can't be there but I know you will be brilliant. Both Bobby and myself are incredibly proud of the fact that, at the tender age of just 71, you are able to follow in the family footsteps and get to play for England. So very proud of you, Tom.' It was read to him as he was about to be interviewed by Sky News. 'It hit me right in the heart,' Tommy tells me. 'I was shocked. I've seen it on the TV and I look like a right plonker because I'm nearly in tears. But that's the way it hit me. I'm choking up now thinking about it. All my life, as long as I can remember, I've respected them two. When they were beginning to be famous, I was only a kid, so I've lived my whole life in their shadow.'

This was Tommy's turn to be the footballer, and it was better late than never. Any chance of a career in the game was ended for Tommy at age 24 when, during a friendly in Widdrington in Northumberland, his kneecap was shattered in a collision with a goalkeeper. 'Oh that was awful,' he recalls. 'I put my hand down and there was no knee. I thought to myself, "Well somebody is going to have to straighten my leg because it is doubled up." So I did it myself. I pushed it back down and the only thing they could find on the football field where we were playing to use as a splint was a corner flag.' Ouch. It meant he never followed his brothers in becoming a professional player, but he is now a proud patron of walking football. He is a representative of The Mature Millers club in Rotherham and plays every Monday and Wednesday. The first rule, of course, is no running. Secondly, the ball is not allowed to go over head height.

Naturally in discussing his brothers' health, the topic of heading crops up. 'I've given it lots of thought and it is so obviously unnatural to head the ball. You aren't designed to have shock like that on your head. That, to me, is painfully obvious. It is so unnatural. My mother had four brothers – Jack, Jim, George and Stan – who all played professional football and were all defenders. They all showed signs of dementia before they died that I saw. I put that down at the time to the very fact that they headed a big, heavy, wet, leather ball on muddy pitches and that couldn't possibly do any good, could it?' Researchers have since suggested the modern ball is as dangerous, if not more because of the speed at which it travels by comparison. 'It's the game we know and love and any sort of change, like non-heading of the ball, would be major. I really don't know the answer.'

Tommy couldn't afford to attend the 1966 World Cup Final. He was 20 years old, working down Lynemouth Colliery and didn't want to trouble Sir Bobby or Jack by asking them to cover his train fare to London. So he cheered them on from afar. Watching *Finding Jack Charlton* was hard for Tommy. 'I could have wept when I saw Jack. I remember him going slightly worse, and slightly worse, and slightly worse. The last time I saw him, his wife brought him here and he hardly knew me. He hardly knew where he was.' Tommy pauses. 'Oh dear. It's very difficult. I watched that and I thought to myself then, "I don't want people to remember our Jack in that state." That wasn't Jack. That was a shell. He should be remembered as what he was – a brilliant, outgoing, intelligent guy. My big brother. His wife, Pat, is a saint. He was well looked-after. You've got to think about people who haven't got anybody like that.' And Sir Bobby? 'Where Jack is ebullient and all the rest of it, Bob is quiet and retiring. A gentleman – gentle being the operative word. Bob wouldn't say boo to a goose. I phone him regularly, and speak to his wife most of the time. Norma is magic. She's done a great job with Bob. She's kept him going.'

Dementia in football wasn't always afforded the recognition it deserved. For too long those with the disease were dismissed as going 'doolally' or 'a bit daft', as they would say in the north-east. Today those terms are recognised as offensive. 'It was in hushed tones,' Tommy concludes. 'Now people talk openly about it. That's what's new. Dementia is not new. If somebody like Bob has dementia, well that's big news, isn't it?' It is, as it was for each of the Boys of '66.

It is no small decision to announce to the world that a loved one is living with dementia. There is no step-by-step how-to guide. Some former footballers can make this call for themselves, like Denis Law, who announced on 19 August 2021 he was the seventh member of Manchester United's 1968 European Cup-winning squad with the disease. 'I do understand what is happening and that is why I want to address my situation now whilst I am able, because I know there will be days when I don't understand and I hate the thought of that right now,' he said. Usually, though, it falls on the family to decide. Some see the benefits of announcing. Others don't.

Sir Geoff Hurst has made up his own mind on whether or not to donate his brain. If his donation can do any good once he's gone then he considers it necessary. 'Absolutely, categorically, yes,' he says. As every World Cup passes, and each group of England players tries and fails to emulate that distant summer, so the scale of the 1966 achievement grows. Before we part ways, I apologise to Sir Geoff for our primarily depressing discussion. He insists it's fine, 'It's a subject which needs addressing. The team spirit was integral to our success. That unity, and the boss at the top who generated that.' Together they brought football home on 30 July 1966. Today manager Sir Alf Ramsey and players Ray Wilson, Martin Peters, Jack Charlton, Nobby Stiles and Sir Bobby Charlton are all united in their own way – by dementia.

# 13

# You Forget, Then You're Forgotten

*Players left for dead and the raw, real human toll
of football's link to dementia*

WALK INTO one dementia-dedicated care home in Worcester
at the start of 2020 and you would be greeted by a wonderful
collection of characters. There was the former fairground worker
shouting 'come on, come on, hook your duck'. There was the old
army major marching up and down the corridor. Then there
was Alf Wood, lovingly known as 'the footballer'. Alf lost a
lot, but never his love of the game he played for Manchester
City, Shrewsbury Town, Millwall and others. He was forever
accompanied by a ball, complete with his name written on it in
permanent marker. He would dribble it down the hallway. He
would shoot it in your direction if you dared jokingly tell him
you were a goalkeeper. That Alf had scoliosis of the spine didn't
stop him. The ladies living in the care home couldn't stop him,
either. They would tell him off, as if he was a kid kicking a ball
in the house and putting the good china at risk. But this man
of football, this icon of the 1960s and '70s with his moustache
and bushy sideburns, this husband to Joan and father to Sam and
Karen would take no notice of their tuts and wagging fingers.

Worcester's specialist dementia unit was Alf's own Wembley,
and he would kick away while whistling the *Match of the Day*
theme tune to himself. Fittingly, that ditty was played at his

funeral, too, after Alf passed away on 10 April 2020 at the age of 74. Covid ultimately claimed Alf, a decade after dementia took hold. The Wood family kindly gave me permission to tell his story, wishing to point out how he was let down by the players' union in later life.

Alf started showing signs of dementia at 58 years old, was diagnosed at 64, moved into the care home at 67, and died at 74. When his family came to collect his possessions from the care home, they found seven tattered balls, and that doesn't include the popped ones discovered hidden under his bed. 'Dad was such a strong man,' says Sam. 'It was his head that went. He didn't have an understanding of who, what, why or where. But he never lost football. He'd put his foot over the top of the ball and kick it back to you. He'd come for you to try to get it through your legs. You could do nothing but cry and laugh. I miss that cheeky man. He adored the carers and they loved him. We couldn't go in because of Covid-19, but the carers told Mum that Dad wouldn't be alone. That meant a lot. He knew he was loved. There were times he'd focus, look at the ball, look at you and then, all in slow motion, he'd swing his leg back. I'd love to know what was going through his head. I'd love to know if all he saw of me was a green shirt with a number one on my back.'

Alf and Joan were childhood sweethearts who married in July 1966, the same month that England were crowned world champions. 'He liked Manchester United as a boy and Mum wasn't happy because she was a City fan,' Sam continues. 'But he did play for City so she forgave him. Dad would whistle along to United songs. For that split second, for that moment you made a connection, that was what the visit to the home was for. Dad was 58 when we started noticing problems. He forgot words very quickly. He'd call a dog a "cow". It went on and on, and got harder and harder. He was 64 when diagnosed with frontotemporal dementia. Mum became a prisoner in her own home and had a breakdown. Dad went into a home at 67 and Mum visited every day. In the early years we'd take him out, until he started trying to open car doors when travelling. Life was hard. But we could have fun with him. We'd play football.'

Sam pauses. It is an upsetting topic, but one which cannot be ignored. 'There was no compassion from the PFA,' she says of the Professional Footballers' Association. 'They didn't want to have the conversation about dementia and football. Old footballers, they were so special, real gentlemen, they played with such passion. There was an aggressiveness on the field but they were gentle giants off it. We have pictures of Dad with blood dripping down from his head and he's still going up to contest a header. His skill was heading and contesting the ball. Later in life you go through such heartache. There's that stress of knowing you have to find £1,000 a week to pay for his care.' Over seven years, that's a bill of roughly £364,000 which needed covering. It's worth remembering at this point that the players' union own 'heritage assets' valued at £10.8m, such as memorabilia, as per their charity's latest accounts filed with Companies House. That includes the L.S. Lowry oil painting *Going To The Match*, purchased at auction in 1999 for £1.9m, close to four times the figure it was expected to command.

Sam says the family received the odd 'small' cheque to cover an expense here and there but they were largely on their own. 'The PFA need to step up and own it. Help people now. Help protect youngsters now. God help us if in the future, we have footballers of the 1990s and 2000s suffering.' The union have improved of late. For all their past sluggishness, they have now created a dementia department, vowing to help former footballers and their families. Their next task is to put this promise into practice; to ensure others aren't left in the same situation as the Woodses were.

Before the end, Alf went through a phase of trying to pull the fire extinguisher off the care home's wall. Then his family realised why. The accompanying warning sign carried the words 'Class A: Wood'. Alf thought it was his name – A. Wood – so figured the extinguisher belonged to him. Also worrying was how this former centre-forward would still try to head the ball in the home. 'That was set in his memory,' explains Sam, who bought a soft foam ball so he could satisfy that urge. Yet the damage was already done back when Alf was playing professionally. Though it took so much from him, the Wood family are glad the game gave him such enjoyment. 'I'm so grateful that football was still so much a part of his life,' says Sam, in tears. 'We have so many memories of him pre-dementia, and so many sad ones after dementia. But football gave us good memories after he was diagnosed, too. As a husband, a dad, a brother, a grandad and great-grandad he was a loving, gentle, caring man. Dementia was a part of his life, but we will never let it take our memories.'

Memories make us who we are. The idea that they shape our identity is the crux of the documentary detailing the life – and near death – of Sir Alex Ferguson. Called *Never Give In*, the film starts with a quiz. 'Test your memory,' says his son and the documentary's director, Jason. Sir Alex is asked on which street he was born in Govan, Glasgow. 'Shieldhall Road.' Correct. He's asked who scored the first goal of his time as Manchester United manager, back in 1986. 'John Sivebæk.' Correct again. He's asked the date of his wedding anniversary to wife Cathy and the birthdates of his three sons, Jason, Darren and Mark. He aces them all. The only question Sir Alex cannot answer is what he remembers of 5 May 2018 – the day a brain haemorrhage almost killed him. 'Nothing,' says this 13-time Premier League title winner. In football, he was the boss. He would select the starting line-up. He would decide the tactics. He would even determine how many minutes should be added on to the end of games – at least that's how the joke goes, hence the term 'Fergie time'. After collapsing, though, he wasn't in charge. He was 76 years old and in the hands of the NHS.

For all that Sir Alex was one of football's most fearsome managers, he had a fear of his own. You learn in this moving documentary it is of losing his lifetime of memories. Jason reveals as much when describing his father's reaction to being told he'd had a bleed on the brain and that he required surgery at Salford Royal Hospital. 'All of a sudden he just put his head in his hands and went, "Ugh, I hope there's nothing wrong with my memory. There better be nothing wrong with my memory." And then he just started telling these random stories where the only connection between any of them was the fact that they all happened a long time ago. I think he's telling me these stories to keep himself convinced that he's still got a memory.' Given an initial 20 per cent chance of survival, he overcame the odds. The operation was a success, though Sir Alex temporarily lost his voice. Doctors handed him a pen and asked him to write down the names of family, friends, footballers he'd managed. Scribbling away, he wrote the same word, over and over. 'Remember.' The thought of descending into a world of his own was Sir Alex's worst nightmare. 'I would have hated to have lost my memory,' the Scot says. 'It would have been a terrible burden on the family. I'm sat in the house and I don't know who I am, I don't know who you are, who my wife is.'

How he grew up in the shadow of the Glaswegian shipyards. How he met Cathy. How in 1978 he took over an Aberdeen team that didn't have a training ground – they used to have to clear the dog muck off the pitch before practising at their local park – and turned them into 1983 European Cup Winners' Cup champions. How he elbowed Celtic and Rangers out of the way and disrupted that duopoly to win three Scottish titles. How he went from being unwanted at Manchester United after his appointment in 1986 – supporters would phone his home to tell him to sod off back to Scotland – to their greatest-ever manager, his most magical night coming in that 1999 Champions League Final against Bayern Munich. Sir Alex's history didn't desert him, mercifully. He couldn't tell you about the brain haemorrhage that almost claimed him that Saturday morning in 2018 but the rest of his memories were safe, still there for rainy day reminiscing.

The opening chapter of this book told the story of another Manchester United great. Charlie Roberts was the former captain who died on 7 August 1939 following a seven-and-a-half-hour operation on the brain. He is buried at St Cross Church cemetery in Clayton, Manchester, a short drive from Old Trafford. It is thanks to the Manchester United Graves Society that we know this. Founded by Iain McCartney, this group have made it their mission to find and, if necessary, restore the final resting place of every player to have pulled on the United shirt. Or the Newton Heath shirt, for that matter, as the club was originally known until 1902. It isn't easy. They aren't simply searching for a Busby Babe. They're looking for the obscure ones, too, like Tom Burke, the painter who died of lead poisoning and whose burial place is proving as elusive as he was down the wing. Considering it is now more than a century since that particular player's passing, problems can only be expected. 'It's pot luck,' says Iain, doing himself a disservice given the work involved.

With each case comes hours upon hours of research and, regrettably on too many occasions, a dead end. If lucky enough to secure an exact location, however, Iain will ask one of the organisation's members to travel to the cemetery for confirmation and a photograph. It isn't always a success story. Sometimes they will find a patch of grass to go with the designated plot number. Sometimes a gravestone crumbling under the weight of time. These are the ones in need of sprucing up, although as Iain has discovered, finding where the person is buried is only half the battle. 'You can't just walk into a cemetery and lay down a new stone,' he says. 'There's a lot of red tape. But I don't think any of these people who played a part in our history should be forgotten.'

Thankfully Charlie Roberts' gravestone is still in good nick, with his proudly proclaiming he captained the club down the road from 1904 to 1913. To date, the Manchester United Graves Society have found 370 graves of former players and managers. Without wishing to make it sound like collecting Panini stickers, Iain considers them 'gots'. The search is never over, however. There are hundreds of others on their list who they still 'need'.

Why do it? 'Because I enjoy it,' explains Iain, a season ticket holder since the 1980s, despite the 12-hour round trip it takes from his home in Dumfries, south-west Scotland. 'Because I'm a supporter. Because it's important to keep the memories of all players alive.' Naturally a worrying number of the men buried in the 370 graves located since the group's launch in 2018 lived then died with dementia. Like David Herd, who is buried in Middlebie, half an hour's drive from Iain's home north of the border. Like Bill Foulkes. Like Tony Dunne. Like Nobby Stiles. Like John Fitzpatrick. All of them were members of the United squad that won the 1968 European Cup, and all of them developed dementia before dying. In his efforts to ensure every representative of United is remembered, Iain has seen how football can forget its lost sons once they are in the ground. It can likewise forget those it's still losing.

The 'forgotten England captain' was how Dave Watson's wife, Penny, described her husband when we first spoke. Dave won 65 caps for England as a strapping central defender who looked like he was chiselled out of stone. His was a full memory bank: of captaining his country; of winning the 1973 FA Cup with Sunderland; of lifting the 1976 League Cup with

Manchester City. Watch back the footage of that '76 final and at full time, you'll see Dave lying down on the doctor's table in the Wembley changing room, his blue City shirt bloodied. He is receiving stitches above his left eye. ITV commentator Brian Moore asks him how it happened. 'It was the back of Alan Gowling's head, actually,' Dave says, live on television and with City physiotherapist Freddie Griffiths standing over him. 'I got a knock early in the first half which bruised it, and then I got another in the second half which opened it up.' Painful? 'No, not really. I've had some local.' Hard as nails, Dave wasn't going to let something as silly as stitches spoil his day at Wembley. 'Tremendous,' he says, sitting up. The Watsons have that shirt from 28 February 1976. It's framed and on display at their family home in Nottingham, bloodstains still visible.

Dave's dementia diagnosis was thrust into the public domain on 7 November 2020 and so was his feeling of abandonment. 'THE FORGOTTEN ENGLAND CAPTAIN' went the headline in the *Daily Mail*, borrowing his wife's description. 'Every day there seems to be something disappearing,' Penny explained in that piece about her 74-year-old partner, who was diagnosed at 68. 'Occasionally I see my Dave. He's still got that wonderful smile. But that person I knew is gone. His spark's gone. It's heartbreaking. We know what the cause is.' It was the years of service he gave the game, she said. Penny is still sure football prompted Dave's downfall and further evidence lies in the family tree. Dave was one of five brothers. Three of them played football to varying levels and – like Dave – Peter and Tony developed neurodegenerative disorders before their deaths. The other two brothers have never been blighted by brain disease. Neither have Dave's three sisters. Only the footballers. The PFA have since acknowledged their attitude towards this problem was nowhere near good enough in the past, and that's welcome news to Penny.

Going public had the desired effect for Dave. He was no longer 'forgotten'. Supporters made sure of that, a post box in the shape of a Sunderland shirt erected outside of the Stadium of Light seeing hundreds of letters written to Dave. It was overwhelming and Penny saw the wholesome side to the game. Looking back now, she's glad they didn't try to hide Dave's diagnosis. 'The players of that era were very proud. Most of them came from humble backgrounds. They had nothing. Somebody who reached the pinnacle – like my Dave did, captaining his country – is not going to go ask for help.' She suspects that is why some players prefer to keep their condition private, 'It's almost like it's a dirty secret. Once you've decided to make it public, accepted it and embraced it, then people should be helping. This is not just for Dave. It's for those down the ladder, too. We didn't make millions from football and we don't live in a mansion. But what about the other guys who didn't even have what we had? What happens with them?'

To answer that, we turn to the tales of two former footballers lost in 2020 – John Haselden and Tommy Carroll. John was the former defender for Rotherham United and Doncaster Rovers who, in the words of his wife Eileen, 'lived a nightmare' up until his death at age 76. 'Hours and hours of going through cupboards and drawers, banging about, lights on, lights off, doors open, doors closed, up and down all night,' Eileen explains. 'He didn't know what he was doing. Clearly, he didn't like me interfering. I used to have to go into the shower with him and he'd be battering me.' This once-loving husband was deemed a risk to himself and to Eileen, so he was sectioned. 'It was awful. They told me he wouldn't be able to come home. They asked me, "How have you coped with him this long?" I just said, "Well, because I love him."' Eileen says football showed 'complete disregard and cowardice' in how it neglected John after she tried to alert the authorities. Ignorance is bliss, says this woman who witnessed the larcenous nature of dementia up close.

As for Tommy, he was the former defender for Ipswich Town and Birmingham City. His gentle nature off the field contrasted with his competitive streak on it. He once played the second half of an Ipswich game away at Chelsea blind in one eye. When his wife, Jean, went looking for him at full time at Stamford Bridge, she learned he had been taken to hospital. Yet after retiring at 32, he started to struggle. His personality changed. He became confused, forgetful, agitated. 'At 57, he had a stroke, and we were told it was cerebrovascular disease – a neurological problem,' says his daughter, Adrienne Fearis. 'That was in 1999 so in 2000, I wrote to the PFA asking for some help in navigating the issues we were experiencing as Dad deteriorated. I believed the cause was Dad's career and damage caused by heading the ball. I wrote to Gordon Taylor, because he was a contemporary of Dad's – they played together at Birmingham – so I thought that he would have been compassionate towards an old colleague. They asked me to fill out a form, which I did, but I never heard anything back. Three years later, when Dad had deteriorated further, I wrote to them again. They asked me to fill out another form and again I heard nothing back.'

Tommy had won 17 caps for the Republic of Ireland so they tried the Football Association of Ireland instead, and received a sympathetic response. 'They treated Dad with the respect that he deserved,' says Adrienne. Tommy died at 77 after spending the last 15 years of his life in full-time care with no support from anyone inside of football. 'The heartbreaking thing is they get this disease so early and are robbed of full and meaningful lives,' Adrienne adds. 'A wife loses a husband, children their dad, grandchildren their grandad.' An autopsy confirmed Tommy had Chronic Traumatic Encephalopathy which, by now, should not be seen as a condition exclusive to American football or boxing.

CTE is infecting football, too, with Brendon Ormsby having been given a tentative diagnosis of the disease. I first met Brendon on 29 October 2019, visiting his home in Selby, North Yorkshire. This former footballer had a whistle and alarm hanging on a lanyard around his neck, and behind him were a series of words Blu-Tacked to the kitchen wall. There was 'Minnie', the name of the Ormsby family dog. 'Wendy', his wife. 'Football', his sport. They were there to assist Brendon after a stroke in 2013 rendered him unable to speak. He had to learn how to talk all over again. Six years later he still could not converse, although the words 'Aston Villa' and 'Leeds United' – two of the clubs he represented so proudly in his prime – seemed to roll off the tongue. 'They're the two things he can say,' said Wendy. Poetic in a way; tragic also.

Brendon was 59 at the time and the wonderful Wendy spoke with such love for her husband, for whom she cared full-time. When she broke into tears, so did he, putting his hand on hers. They had been together for 45 years and were childhood sweethearts. 'He would head the ball if it was two feet off the ground,' Wendy explained, providing an insight into the type of wholehearted player Brendon was. 'An old-fashioned centre-half. He'd stay for hours after a training session to practise heading. When he was younger, he never used to moan to me. But I was talking to Gary Williams – a former team-mate of Brendon's – and he said when he was at Villa he got headaches. I want to stress: Brendon loved football and still loves football. He went into non-league because he loved it that much, but he had to stop playing because he got detached retinas. Boxers get that. Even then we had to force him. He used to run the ex-Leeds players' matches – he knew he couldn't head the ball but sometimes he couldn't help himself. We'd go mad.'

Brendon's most memorable moment in a Leeds shirt came in the FA Cup's fifth round on 21 February 1987. Facing First

Division side Queens Park Rangers, his winner at Elland Road ensured the Second Division hosts were through to the quarter-finals. It was a thumping header, too. Back post. Bang. One step closer to Wembley. After finishing football, Brendon held five jobs – he was a postman, Elland Road tour guide, Press Association reporter, *Yorkshire Evening Post* columnist and coach for Leeds. Yet now, he was reliant on his wife.

His deterioration had a detrimental impact on Wendy. Her hair started to fall out, having developed alopecia due to stress. She was exhausted. She still is, with Brendon worsening and Wendy continuing to care for him. Visits to their neurologist in York led to Brendon being diagnosed with probable CTE. 'He's too vulnerable to be left on his own. He'd go off on his bike and come back covered in mud. I'd ask, "What did you do?" And he didn't know. He'd take the dog for a walk and come back soaking wet. He'd been in the river. I know I can't leave him on his own, because I cannot trust what he does. Anybody who is in a caring role, you find it really difficult to ask for help. It's just so difficult.' Going cap in hand isn't easy. There's a guilt attached to it.

Football cannot escape its lack of compassion. There are too many sorry stories like Alf Wood's, Dave Watson's, John Haselden's, Tommy Carroll's and Brendon Ormsby's for the game to say otherwise. It can only ensure it changes its ways so that footballers don't continue to feel forgotten. This book began with a foreword from Chris Sutton about his father, Mike, who played professionally and died aged 76 after a decade of living with dementia. That was the son's perspective. We end with the wife's.

The following is an account written by Mike's other half, Josephine, describing the hell on earth that she and her husband endured. She penned these personal thoughts a month before he passed away on 26 December 2020.

## 11 November 2020

My Mike was a proud man. If he had any realisation of what dementia has reduced him to now, I know he would feel humiliated. When we met in 1964, football was Mike's life. He was playing for his hometown club Norwich City, having left school at 15 to pursue a career as a professional. After cruciate ligament damage at 27, Mike attended Loughborough University, earning a double first-class honours degree in biology and physical education. He became a PE teacher, and was always so kind to those who had not had the best of luck in life. Mike knew how to get the best out of his students, who respected him so. He ran extracurricular activities, coached for Norwich and was a wonderful father to Ian, Rachel, Lucy, John and Chris, too.

Now 76, he is in a care home, nearing the end. Other families in similar situations to ours will recognise the stages of Mike's regression since 2010. There was general forgetfulness; failing to remember family and friends' names and normally familiar routes when driving, cycling and walking. Sudden and irrational loss of temper; shouting, throwing things, punching walls and doors. Mike was persuaded to see a doctor who banned him from driving. He'd been diagnosed with dementia, and I had to sell the car as he kept insisting he could drive. We went to see a specialist who said he had severe frontal and temporal lobe damage – caused by heading balls and blows to the head. He was told, 'You are not the first professional footballer to come through that door and you won't be the last.' This was in 2014.

The fits of temper increased and with them the use of bad language. The outside doors had to be double-locked to stop Mike from going out and getting lost. The kitchen door was locked at night to prevent him from touching taps and appliances in case I didn't hear him get up. He would follow me around all day long as I was doing housework or cooking – it seemed he needed to know I was always close by. He became delusional and paranoid, thinking there were other people in our home. Mike was not able to find the toilet, so during the night I'd set an alarm for 1.30am, 4am and 6am to take him. Even so, I would find puddles of urine in different places. I had to become a kind of 'mother' figure to Mike as he didn't know how to wash or dress himself.

Everything became so wearisome. I feared for my own sanity and had suicidal thoughts at times, so we could finish our lives together. He used to love writing in his diary. Then one day, he found he didn't know how to use a pen and never wrote another word. We used to play cribbage. Again, one day we were playing and the next he told me he never had before. He retained his physical skills. When playing short tennis, he never hit a ball out of court or into the net! But when looking at photographs, Mike might recognise himself in his younger days, but not himself when older.

The agitation and aggression began to be directed at me, and our children insisted that it was time for Mike to go into care. I felt I was abandoning him. It is heartbreaking having to leave a loved one behind in a care home. Mike is well looked-after – his amazing carers are so kind to him – but it has come at a price.

Savings have almost disappeared to cover costs. In March, before the initial lockdown, he still had a life, seeing family and friends, being with others in the home's coffee shop and going out for walks, playing table tennis. The rules which 'officialdom' have placed on care homes has reduced him now to lying in bed, with a loss of mobility which will never return.

I am the only one allowed to visit, and that is very hard for our family and friends who have not set eyes on Mike since 16 March. I would like my husband to be at home with me, his family and friends for the little time he has left. I tried to make that happen. Mike cannot walk anymore, and I hoped he might spend his final days looking out on the garden of the home we shared for more than four decades. But the reality is two qualified carers have to be on call at all times for his complicated nursing needs. So it is in the care home where we will ultimately lose Mike without his family and friends getting to say a proper goodbye.

**Josephine Sutton**

The raw, real human toll. Mike died in that care home 45 days later. Chris says his dad had Chronic Traumatic Encephalopathy and he considers that to be cold, hard evidence that his death was a consequence of his career. Football is an emotional game. It's the highs of winning, lows of losing and everything in between. It's the drama of a player coming back to haunt his former club and celebrating when he scores, all sentimentality tossed aside. It's the hilarity of a striker slicing a shot so wide that it flies out for a throw-in, followed by chants of, 'What the f***ing hell was that?' It's the butterflies in your stomach as you enter the stadium, the rousing roar at kick-off and the euphoria of a stoppage-time winner. It's beautiful. And yet there's no beauty in what Josephine just described. There is an ugly side to this game of 11 v 11, and unfortunate losers among those who spent their lives trying to be winners.

# Bibliography

**Newspapers, magazines and websites**
*Daily Mail*
*Mail on Sunday*
*Daily Telegraph* and *Sunday Telegraph*
*The Times* and *Sunday Times*
*Daily Express*
*Daily Mirror* and *Sunday Mirror*
*Daily Star*
*The Guardian*
*The Observer*
*The Sun*
*The Independent*
*New York Times*
*TIME*
*Soccer Review*
*Football League Review*
*FIFA Magazine*
*Sports Journalists' Association*
talkSPORT
*The Athletic*
The Press Association
*The Herald*
*Dundee Evening Telegraph*
*Lincolnshire Echo*
*Birmingham Mail*
*Barnsley Chronicle*
*Newcastle Journal*
*Liverpool Echo*
*Daily Post*

*Northern Daily Telegraph*
*Burnley Express*
*Hull Daily Mail*
*Gloucester Citizen*
*Belfast Telegraph*
*La Gazzetta dello Sport*
*The Age*
ESPN
*Air Force Magazine*
Concussion Legacy Foundation
Boston University
The Jeff Astle Foundation
PINK Concussions
The Drake Foundation
The Glasgow Brain Injury Research Group
England Football Online
*Ottawa Citizen*
Concussion in Sport Group
The Premier League
The Football Association
UEFA
FIFA
*National Collegiate Athletic Association medical handbook for
    schools and colleges*
The British Newspaper Archive
CBC News

## Books
Bent, I., McIlroy, R., Mousley, K., Walsh, P., *Football
    Confidential* (BBC Worldwide Publishing, 1999)
Calvin, M., *State of Play: Under the Skin of the Modern Game*
    (Arrow Books, 2019)
Cox, M., *The Mixer: The Story of Premier League Tactics, from
    Route One to False Nines* (HarperCollins, 2017)
Cullis, S., *All For The Wolves* (Rupert Hart-Davis, 1960)
Fainaru, S., Fainaru-Wada, M., *League of Denial: The
    NFL, Concussions, and the Battle for Truth* (Three
    Rivers Press, 2013)

Giller, N., *Danny Blanchflower: This WAS His Life: The story Eamonn Andrews could not tell* (Norman Giller Publishing, 2014)

Hill, B., *My Gentleman Jim: A Love Story* (Book Guild Publishing, 2015)

Hughes, C., *The Winning Formula: Soccer Skills and Tactics* (William Collins Sons & Co, 1990)

McIlvanney, H., *McIlvanney on Football* (Mainstream Publishing, 1994)

Nowinski, C., *Head Games: Football's Concussion Crisis from the NFL to Youth Leagues* (Drummond Publishing Group, 2006)

Phillips, Dr N., *Doctor to the World Champions: My Autobiography* (Trafford Publishing, 2009)

Ruddock, N., *Hell Razor: The Autobiography of Neil Ruddock* (Collins Willow, 1999)

Sutton, C., *You're Better Than That! How to Fix Modern Football* (Monoray, 2020)

Tatum, J., *They Call Me Assassin* (Avon Books, 1980)

Various, *The Football Association Book for Boys* (The Naldrett Press, 1949)

Wilson, J., *Inverting The Pyramid: The History of Football Tactics* (Orion, 2008)

## Film and television

*Concussion* (Peter Landesman)
*Fantasy Football League*
*Finding Jack Charlton* (Gabriel Clarke, Pete Thomas)
*Head Games: The Global Concussion Crisis* (Steve James)
*Match of the Day*
*Monday Night Raw*
*Monty Python's The Meaning of Life* (Terry Jones)
*Raging Bull* (Martin Scorsese)
*Sir Alex Ferguson: Never Give In* (Jason Ferguson)
Footage from Amazon Prime, BBC, BT Sport, Bundesliga, ESPN, FIFA, Fox Sports, ITV, Netflix, Premier League, Sky Sports, UEFA, YouTube

## Radio
BBC Radio 5 Live
talkSPORT

## Statistics
Opta
Squawka

## Scientific articles

Autti, T, et al, 'Brain lesions in players of contact sports', *The Lancet* (1997)

Casper, Stephen, et al, 'Toward Complete, Candid, and Unbiased International Consensus Statements on Concussion in Sport', *Journal of Law, Medicine & Ethics* (2021)

Harrison, Martland, 'Punch Drunk', *Journal of the American Medical Association* (1928)

Hawkins, RD, et al, 'The association football medical research programme: an audit of injuries in professional football', *British Journal of Sports Medicine* (2001)

Hof, Patrick, et al, 'Neuropathological observations in a case of autism presenting with self-injury behaviour', *Acta Neuropathol* (1991)

Ietswaart, Magdalena, 'Evidence for Acute Electrophysiological and Cognitive Changes Following Routine Soccer Heading', *eBioMedicine* (2016)

Lindsay KW, et al, 'Serious Head Injury in Sport', *British Medical Journal* (1980)

Manley, Geoff, et al, 'A systematic review of potential long-term effects of sport-related concussion', *British Journal of Sports Medicine* (2017)

Matser, JT, et al, 'Chronic traumatic brain injury in professional soccer players', *Neurology* (1998)

Matthews, WB, 'Footballer's migraine', *British Medical Journal* (1972)

McCrory, Paul, et al, 'Consensus statement on concussion in sport—the 5th international conference on concussion in sport held in Berlin, October 2016', *British Journal of Sports Medicine* (2017)

McKee, Ann, et al, 'Chronic Traumatic Encephalopathy in athletes: progressive tauopathy after repetitive head injury', *Journal of Neuropathology and Experimental Neurology* (2009)

McKee, Ann, et al, 'Clinicopathological Evaluation of Chronic Traumatic Encephalopathy in Players of American Football', *Journal of the American Medical Association* (2017)

McKee, Ann, et al, 'Duration of American Football Play and Chronic Traumatic Encephalopathy', *Annals of Neurology* (2019)

McKee, Ann, et al, 'The spectrum of disease in Chronic Traumatic Encephalopathy', *Brain* (2013)

Mez, Jesse, et al, 'Structural MRI profiles and tau correlates of atrophy in autopsy-confirmed CTE', *Alzheimer's Research & Therapy* (2021)

Millspaugh, JA, 'Dementia pugilistica', *US Naval Med Bull* (1937)

Omalu, Bennet, et al, 'Chronic traumatic encephalopathy in a National Football League player', *Neurosurgery* (2005)

Nauman, Eric, et al, 'Collegiate women's soccer players suffer greater cumulative head impacts than their high school counterparts', *Journal of Biomechanics* (2015)

Randolph, Christopher, 'Chronic traumatic encephalopathy is not a real disease', *Archives of Clinical Neuropsychology* (2018)

Randolph, Christopher, 'Is Chronic Traumatic Encephalopathy a Real Disease?' *Current Sports Medicine Reports* (2014)

Roberts, GW, et al, 'Dementia in a punch-drunk wife', *The Lancet* (1990)

Sanderson, Jimmy, et al, 'I Was Able to Still Do My Job on the Field and Keep Playing: An Investigation of Female and Male Athletes' Experiences With (Not) Reporting Concussions', *Communication and Sport* (2017)

Slobounov, Semyon, et al, 'Alteration of posture-related cortical potentials in mild traumatic brain injury', *Neuroscience Letters* (2005)

Smith, Douglas, et al, 'Newfound sex differences in axonal structure underlie differential outcomes from in vitro traumatic axonal injury', *Experimental Neurology* (2018)

Smith, Gordon, Pell, Jill, 'Parachute use to prevent death and major trauma related to gravitational challenge: systematic review of randomised controlled trials', *British Medical Journal* (2003)

Sortland O, Tysvaer AT, 'Brain damage in former association football players', *Neuroradiology* (1989)

Spear, Jon, 'Are Professional Footballers at Risk of Developing Dementia?', *International Journal of Geriatric Psychiatry* (1995)

Stewart, Walter F, et al, 'Heading Frequency Is More Strongly Related to Cognitive Performance Than Unintentional Head Impacts in Amateur Soccer Players', *Frontiers in Neurology* (2018)

Stewart, Willie, et al, 'Association of Sex With Adolescent Soccer Concussion Incidence and Characteristics', *JAMA Network Open* (2021)

Stewart, Willie, et al, 'Association of Field Position and Career Length With Risk of Neurodegenerative Disease in Male Former Professional Soccer Players', *JAMA Neurology* (2021)

Stewart, Willie, et al, 'Chronic Traumatic Encephalopathy is a common co-morbidity, but less frequent primary dementia in former soccer and rugby players', *Acta Neuropathologica* (2019)

Stewart, Willie, et al, 'Primum non nocere: a call for balance when reporting on CTE', *The Lancet* (2019)

Stewart, Willie, et al, 'Neurodegenerative Disease Mortality among Former Professional Soccer Players', *The New England Journal of Medicine* (2019)

Tierney, Gregory, et al, 'Force experienced by the head during heading is influenced more by speed than the mechanical properties of the football', *Scandinavian Journal of Medicine & Science in Sports* (2020)

Tysvaer, AT, Løchen EA, 'Soccer injuries to the brain: A neuropsychologic study of former soccer players', *The American Journal of Sports Medicine* (1991)

Tysvaer, AT, Storli, O-V, 'Soccer injuries to the brain: A neurologic and electroencephalographic study of active football players', *The American Journal of Sports Medicine* (1989)

191

Williams DJ, Tannenberg, AE, 'Dementia pugilistica in an alcoholic achondroplastic dwarf', *Pathology* (1996)

Wüllenweber, R, 'Über Verletzungen des Nervensystems beim Fußballspiel', *Deutsche Medizinische Wochenschrift* (1962)